"Taking on the gift of an unwanted experience and healing your soul—that's what Vanessa Broers did with motherhood. She shows us how (with courage and a steadfast commitment) we can begin the undoing and maturing that brings us back home to what we really are. Packed with real-ness, truth, and hard-fought wisdom, Vanessa's book challenges us all to do the work of becoming fully whole, and human, beings of love. An honest, beautiful, heart-expanding must-read!"

—MELISSA FORD
Author of *Living Service: The Journey of a Prosperous Coach*

"Vanessa Broers has written a poetic and deeply personal book about motherhood that is also about acceptance, love, courage, and joy. If you want your heart touched, and your spirit lifted, this book will do it."

—STEVE CHANDLER
Author of *Time Warrior*

"*We Are One* is an extraordinary story of love and loving oneself, the love of a child, loving one's spouse, and accepting what is. Through this journey the reader gets a glimpse of Vanessa's powerful dedication to her own path of discovery and to the deep service she provides her clients. She holds nothing back. Highly recommended!"

—KAMIN SAMUEL
Author of *Successful Life Transformation Journal: How to Create Success on Your Own Terms*

"In this book, Vanessa shares her beautiful, and at times harrowing journey of motherhood to show us what transformation looks and feels like. In every chapter she allows us to open our hearts *with* her through each story she shares. Profound wisdom and thoughtful questions are sprinkled throughout the book, which I love because it's so much more than motherhood and partnership she's describing here. She had me laughing out loud because I recognized myself as a young mother trying to figure out who I was separate and connected to my girls, fumbling and bumbling and trying to do what I thought was best. I also had tears of joy as I witnessed her expanding into the huge space of love that exists when you surrender to the unpredictable beauty of life. What a delight it is to read a mother's journey, really a woman's journey, into waking up to who she really is."

—TINA QUINN
Author of *Invisible Things: The most important things in life are the ones you can't see*

"In a sea of self-promoting self-help books, Vanessa's writing is a salvation from mundane study of self-improvement, delivering us back into the joy of reading. While she indeed delivers a depth of insight that is transcendent of the common narrative, she does so with the grace of an award-winning novelist. What fun it is to be laughing out loud while reading and to be learning new ways to think about ourselves and our life while looking forward to every paragraph. This is simply great writing—a page-turner filled with diamonds for a better life."

—JOHN PATRICK MORGAN
Philosopher and Champion for Being

"*We Are One* completely spoke to my heart. In her inspiring book, Vanessa Broers holds nothing back in this beautiful tribute to her daughter, Pepper. Her engaging stories about her own rebirth into motherhood are incredibly relatable, and full of pearls of wisdom. Her stories brought me back to many of my own experiences of motherhood: the depth of love, the choices, and the messiness. This is a must-read for women who are searching for self-love, inner peace, and complete acceptance."

—KAREN DAVIS

Co-author of *Unconventional Wisdom, When All Boats Rise, and How to Get the Most Out of Coaching*

"This book is a gift. Vanessa held nothing back and pulled no punches; she narrates her truth because she writes for her soul. That's the gift. This book will strike a chord in all of us touched by motherhood, sisterhood, or daughterhood. *We Are One* is Vanessa's hero's journey—it can be as acutely distressing as it is pleasurable, and as totally exhausting as it is insightful. Her journey is not your typical motherhood tale but instead one of intense self-inquiry, discovery, and joy. Buckle up!"

—MARI CARMEN PIZARRO

Author of *The High Energy Body: 7 Strategies to Optimize Your Energy, Eat Smarter and Live Longer*

"This book is fantastic! Vanessa beautifully articulates the raw, real, rich experience of being a new mom, a coach, a wife, a human in all its complexity—and shares it in a way that is tangible and relatable. I laughed and cried while reading it. The microscopic truth she tells often put words to experiences I've had but could not describe.

"I felt seen. I felt inspired throughout, and through her vulnerability, I felt truly connected to the beauty of my human self but also to the depth of wisdom present in my soul. This is a wonderful read I highly recommend. An absolute page-turner."

—AILA COATS
Author of *Coaching Teens Well*

We Are One

By Vanessa Broers

Cover design by Skyler Kratofil.

Published by

◀ köehlerbooks ™

3705 Shore Drive
Virginia Beach, VA 23455
800–435–4811
www.koehlerbooks.com

WE ARE ONE

HOW ONE WOMAN RECLAIMED HER IDENTITY THROUGH MOTHERHOOD

Vanessa Broers

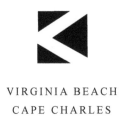

VIRGINIA BEACH
CAPE CHARLES

This book is for Pepper, whose surprise entry into my life saved my life.

And to my mother: If all women had children, and sooner, we'd spend a lot less time blaming our own mothers.

To Sibe, for always allowing me to share our life to teach. And for sharing your life with me.

And to all women. Children or not, your love is so big, you have the capacity to love the whole world.

TABLE OF CONTENTS

1.

CHEWING ON BONES

I KNOW PAIN INTIMATELY. Betrayal (as both the betrayed and betrayer), rejection, anger, defeat, loss, grief, disappointment, sadness, and the madness of primal rage. The kind of pain that would make you ferociously dig up graves in a cemetery and start chewing on the bones. If you can't totally relate to that metaphor without cringing at my insanity, then you've never felt the kind of rage I'm talking about. And if you have? Well then, have a seat, my friend. Plenty of bones to go around.

I know the territory completely. I've been lost there for decades at a time. I know every detour, every dead end, every insidiously mismarked trailhead that promises freedom but predestines you to loop back on yourself and start again at the beginning, getting infinitely lost in the maze.

I was close to pain for a long time. Knowing me, you might never see it, but I felt its presence constantly lurking in the depths of my being, threatening to swallow me if I let my guard down for one second. As a result, I spent years with a clenched feeling in my solar plexus that I refused to call anxiety but which was, in fact, making me very anxious. I couldn't sit still. I had to be moving constantly. This manifested as an eating and exercise disorder in college, a travel disorder in my twenties (also known as backpacking), and most recently as a productivity disorder.

But I have spent the last fifteen years studying the maps of pain and suffering and have started to understand the territory. Luckily, though I didn't see it initially, life presented me with the opportunity to dissolve completely into my pain and emerge on the other side—free, peaceful, and *me* for the first time in my life. It allowed me to understand my pain and leave my suffering behind in the process.

Now the once confusing maze, which was impossible to navigate and even more impossible to escape, is a completely organized mess. Complex but actually quite simple to navigate and escape when you understand it. I see the subtle differentiations between roads; I get that the territory of pain is filled with mirages, quicksand, and trick exits. I see now that with the right knowledge, resolve, and support, not only is it possible to part ways with suffering as your shadow, you can experience compassion for it, even gratitude and a sweet nostalgia for its presence as you leave it behind for good.

2.

WHAT I DON'T WANT YOU TO KNOW

I NEVER WANTED to be a mother.

God, it feels so wrong to say that.

Partly because I feel like we're not supposed to say that. And partly because I love my daughter so much that it would kill me if she interpreted that as her being unwanted. (🍼, I love you, and you're the best thing that ever happened to me.) I didn't want to be a mother because I had based my entire identity around not being *my* mother.

The best way to not be *my* mother was to not be *a* mother.

I had so much anger toward my mother from my childhood that I had been running from it my entire life. I tried to succeed my way out of painful life experiences that ended more than two decades ago.

I spent much of my pregnancy letting go of that anger. My mom and I have always been close; I just didn't realize that I was still holding so much anger toward her. I started to see how my annoyance and impatience with her came from that residual anger. Through letting go, I have been able to see how great my mother is and the incredible gifts I have received from her. I feel closer, more accepting, and much more understanding than I did before.

I'd be honored to model her selflessness, generosity, and limitless heart. (*Ho'ponopono*, Mom.)

Before Pepper, I'd spent the previous ten years pouring every ounce of my energy into creating a successful life-coaching practice and establishing myself as a professional coach. Motherhood was never in the cards for me. And while I can honestly say that I have enjoyed every moment of motherhood so far, I am blown away by the complexity and depth of it. The experience has been an incredible challenge of surrender and self-awareness in order to move through the difficulty of not only splitting my time and energy but also evolving my identity to fit this new, unexpected life.

This book is meant to capture the first year of this massive experience and my challenge to *expand* into this sacred role and use it to expand in all areas of my life.

These essays share the raw, real, and in-the-moment complexities of expanding into motherhood, career, and love instead of contracting into a default conditioned future of resentment, disconnection, and divisiveness.

3.

"YOU'RE F*CKING PREGNANT, VANESSA."

"I'M NOT FEELING THIS TACO. My appetite has been weird since my work with my shaman," I said to my friend Claire while sipping a margarita on a Tuesday night. "I'm just not craving crappy food anymore. I'm not digging eggs and I can't drink coffee. Gross," I added as I threw down my chorizo taco. "Sausage either."

Claire paused, amused. I saw the almost invisible turn of the corner of her mouth. Before putting her taco into her mouth she said, "You're fucking pregnant, Vanessa," then bit into her taco, never looking up.

I told her to go fuck herself and moved on to the queso.

The next morning, I bailed on our morning workout in a text exchange.

ME: *I can't get out of bed before eight am. I think it's the time change.*
CLAIRE: *Vanessa. The one hour time change? You.are.pregnant*
ME: 👆

Later that week, we were at the grocery store, and Claire met me at the checkout with a pregnancy test.

I was so sure I wasn't pregnant that I took it from her just to shut her up (and secretly had purchased one of my own), and went home to take it.

I had a coaching call with a client in twenty minutes—more than enough time to put this to rest.

Except . . . I was fucking pregnant.

I threw the test reflexively and walked out of the bathroom. A few minutes later I went back in, searching under my sink for wherever it had landed.

I was fucking pregnant. And I didn't have health insurance. And I had an IUD in. *And* I had a coaching call in fifteen minutes.

I sat waiting for my call to start in a trancelike state of disbelief. A small dam, holding strong for decades, had given way somewhere in my subconscious, and a terrifying awareness flooded my entire being.

The moment I discovered I was pregnant was also the moment I discovered that I did not want children.

I had convinced myself that I would want them someday. I always told myself that I just wasn't ready. I set different milestones for when it would make more sense. In that surreal moment, I realized that day would have never come.

I sat back in my throne-style, green-velvet chair and closed my eyes. *It's okay*, I thought. *I have spent the past two years working on letting go of control and practicing surrender. I can surrender to this too.* I lied to myself and ignored the subtle sinking sensation in my gut.

Years before, a friend of mine became pregnant with an IUD and had to terminate the pregnancy because it was unsafe. For a moment, I hoped I would have to as well. I felt a tiny bit of relief.

Somehow (I like to believe it was a testament to my dedication to practicing presence), I made it through a two-hour coaching call. It was 11:30 a.m.

When I hung up, I called Sibe, who wasn't supposed to be home until nine that night. The moment he answered the phone, he knew something was up.

"What's wrong?" he asked before I said anything other than "Hello." "I can hear it in your voice."

Sibe has a psychic-level awareness of even the slightest variance in someone's energy. It's impossible to hide anything from him. Even when you think you have successfully hidden something from yourself, he can sense it. There are some mornings that I'll have woken up but haven't even opened my eyes, still lying with my back to him, and he will roll over and anxiously demand, "What's wrong?" Which will scare the shit out of me, because it's not until I'm surprised by his anxious demand that I even know he's awake. It won't be until he asks that I become aware of a microscopic sense of anxiousness in me that is likely the remnant feeling of an odd dream or the subconscious awareness that I forgot to respond to an email.

I didn't want to tell him that I was pregnant over the phone, but despite my efforts to try to throw the hound dog off my scent, it was pointless. An episode from *Full House* came to mind, when Aunt Becky spends the entire day preparing a meal of baby foods to create a fun, surprise guessing game to announce her pregnancy to Uncle Jesse.

This would be the first of many realizations that the reality of this journey was not going to play out like a perfectly scripted sitcom.

"I'm pregnant."

He told me much later that the moment those words came out of my mouth, the biggest smile ever came over his face.

He had four clients that day and I had two more.

Within the next fifteen minutes, every single one of them canceled.

4.

IS MY LOVE REALLY BIG ENOUGH?

I WAS LYING IN BED last night looking at Sibe, and wanting to be looking at Pepper—just a few weeks old—instead. He was sleeping, and I lay there feeling distant from him and saw a possible default future unfolding in front of me.

There's such an indescribably strong, primal connection to your child, such a deep love and an evolutionary, all-encompassing compulsion to be looking at, touching, holding, and thinking about them constantly.

I was prepared for this. I was unprepared for the painful distance it would create in my heart for Sibe.

No, that's not true. I was completely unprepared for the intense love I had for my kid and terrified that a child would create distance between Sibe and me. I was both prepared for and afraid of that.

In that moment, I could see how easily women fall into the default future. They go from wives to mothers. Their lover turns into their helper. I become the main caregiver of Pepper, know her intuitively and intimately, and Sibe becomes my support person. I feel less connected to him and more interested in spending time with Pepper. I don't mean to, but tiny moments like this one in bed compound over time. And over time, we grow apart.

I also happen to know a thing about default futures: they are only default if you do nothing.

Last night I became acutely aware of my challenge: how to be a wife AND a mother. How can I be a wife and mother and ME—and a professional coach who loves herself, her life, her kid, her career, and her husband?

I know love in and of itself is big enough to hold all of these aspects of life and that things will evolve to get easier. Life will become more normal and less overwhelming, but right then, it felt like *my* love wasn't big enough. Like I didn't have enough to go around.

Tears silently fell down my cheeks while Sibe slept, unaware that any of this was going on. I decided in that moment I must figure out how to expand my love to be big enough to swallow everything.

5.

EVERYTHING I'VE EVER WORKED FOR

AFTER SEEING THE DOCTOR and finding out that everything was in the right place (including the IUD that I had sworn was now somewhere in my stomach), we were on track to have this baby. Sibe was thrilled.

At first, I felt pretty peaceful about it. It also seemed pretty magical that I really didn't have a say in being pregnant, creating a connection to a bigger life force.

But there was a growing whisper. One that I ignored. A subtle lack of excitement mixed with a little dread and then layered with guilt. Guilt that Sibe was so excited and I wasn't. Guilt that a great friend of mine was desperately trying to have a baby, and here I was, gifted with one, and ungrateful and upset about it. Not wanting people to know that I was pregnant because I felt ashamed and worried about how they'd look at me. And confused. Where was all of this coming from?

I felt too guilty and ashamed of my reaction to share it with anyone. Layered onto that, I felt terrified that my baby would feel all of this and feel unwanted. So I stuffed it down.

Sibe kept asking if I was okay. I kept minimizing how I felt. Not just to him, but to myself.

A week later, in a session with our coach, I completely broke down. Sobbing. In one breath, I confessed that I was terrified that it felt like everything I'd ever worked for was being taken away from me. I confessed that I wanted to be a high-level executive coach, not a mother. After a week of telling him I was okay, the words I said were cutting, unexpected, and incredibly painful for Sibe to hear. Unsurprisingly, they created doubt in him over whether I wanted this baby, and he was hurt and upset. To me, his response validated the guilt I felt for having these feelings that was causing me to suppress how I felt in the first place.

While it was true that I realized I never would have chosen to have kids, I was very clear that I was going to have this one.

While it was true that I want to be a high-level executive coach, I knew deeper down that the baby wasn't necessarily going to take that away.

But Sibe didn't know that I knew that. He heard me say I was okay and then witnessed me have a complete breakdown.

About a week later, in a session with my shaman, he opened by saying, "I bet it feels like everything you've ever worked for is being taken away from you." He paused. "That's because it is. This pregnancy is life's gift to you. Your entire identity is built around escaping your childhood. It's too small, it lacks spiritual depth, and this pregnancy is designed to systematically destroy the identity you've created so you can expand into who you're meant to be."

6.

MY NEXT BOYFRIEND WILL LOVE COUNTRY MUSIC

AT THE END OF THE SEPTEMBER before I knew I was pregnant, I had my annual tarot reading with my tarot lady, Leslie. I was satisfied until the very end when Leslie casually added, as she was shuffling her cards back into the deck, "By the way, your womb is getting ready for a baby."

"Yeah, right," I laughed. I shared this absurdity with my friends over cocktails just after my reading, all of us laughing at the unlikely thought of me with a kid.

I was pregnant by the middle of October.

In another reading with Leslie the following January, I couldn't stop crying. I don't know if it was pregnancy hormones or what, but I left a yoga class in tears that morning, heard a baby cry on my way out, and power-walked to my car just in time for my tears to explode. By the time I got to my reading, I had been crying the entire day. I even called Sibe laughing, at one point, because I couldn't stop crying.

"This baby is coming to heal you," Leslie said as she read my cards.

In working closely with my shaman during my pregnancy, I slowly began to understand my resistance to becoming a mother. Some of it had to do with the anger I had toward my own mother. Some of it was unresolved emotion from difficult moments in my childhood. Some of it came from lives long before this one.

But most of it was because becoming a mother really shattered how I saw myself fitting into the world—as a badass professional coach who slayed life and made shit happen. Being a mother would ruin all of that. I didn't want to split my focus. I didn't want to take my eyes off my career for a second. I didn't want my heart divided. I had poured my entire sense of self into conquering the world through coaching. And almost instantly, this little grain of rice crumbled that entire structure.

I was devastated, confused, and angry, and it took me my entire pregnancy and the deepest work I'd ever done on myself to learn to let go of everything I thought I was and open up space to become a professional coach *and* kick-ass mom. I had to learn to trust life, which was a phrase I intellectually understood but couldn't bring myself to actually do.

For most of my life, I felt like I was running down a street that was crumbling under my feet, my foot landing just seconds before the road fell away beneath it.

I could never stop running. Having a child felt like coming to a grinding halt while the ground disappeared and I fell into a painful, infinite oblivion.

But month by month and session by session, I started to heal. And as I began to understand why I was the way I was and mend the effects of painful life experiences I had suppressed for thirty years, my inner world calmed down.

I no longer felt the contraction in my solar plexus that I called anxiety. Productivity no longer equated to safety. My sense of security stopped being measured by the number of dollars in my bank account. (And thank god for that because I imploded my business during this time.)

As I'm writing this, it's 5:30 a.m. and I'm lying in bed, sandwiched between a sleeping Pepper and a sleeping Opi (my huge mastiff)— the duo I've now started calling PepperOpi.

Pepper started crying in her sleep, and it was the sweetest, most heartbreaking little cry. I immediately put my hands under her head to cradle her and kissed her forehead to let her know I was there, and her cry faded into a whimper as she fell back to sleep.

I felt so much love for her in that moment. But I was also aware of a subtle sense of pride, which caught my attention. It wasn't pride like "I'm so proud of Pepper." It was more of a "Hey, look at me and how great I'm doing." I observed a thought: *I'm going to make sure you always feel safe and you know I'm strong and always have your back.* While on the surface there's nothing wrong with this thought, it occurred to me that wanting to feel safe and know that someone had my back was *my* thing, not Pepper's. This is a problem for two reasons.

First, in trying to overcorrect for what I wanted and felt I didn't have, I might miss what she actually needs. How do I know if Pepper wants or needs me to be strong and prove the world is safe? So far, she has no reason to believe it isn't. And in my valiant attempts to curate a world where she has nothing to worry about, I might miss her requests to be seen for who *she* is in whatever expression and form that shows up.

I envisioned Pepper crying to be celebrated for who she is while I'm yelling, "Don't you see?! The world is safe!" And she's yelling back, "Yeah, I know! Help me figure out how to make friends!" But I can't hear her requests over my own triumph.

Of course, none of this happens consciously. But I believe it's why all of us on some level blame our parents for our own unmet needs. Without the awareness of this, we project our own needs onto our kids, and miss their requests.

We do this to our children, our partners, our health, finances, and careers.

In high school, I had a major crush on a guy. He was angsty, artsy, and loved R&B. And he broke my heart. So my seventeen-year-old heart made a declaration: "The next guy I date will love country music." And he did. The next guy I dated loved country music. This guy also broke my heart, but at least he didn't listen to R&B.

While seemingly ridiculous, this *is* actually what we do in all areas of our life. We jump from boyfriend to boyfriend, job to job, from our role as daughter to mother, trying to make up for the inadequacies of our previous experience by projecting its opposite onto our future desires and current circumstances.

The second problem is that I might be successful in creating a safe world for Pepper but end up disappointed or even resentful when Pepper doesn't appreciate the world I created for her that she never asked for.

When we were preparing for Pepper's arrival, Sibe and I admittedly lost our minds. We bought a Pottery Barn nursing chair and "woodland" shelf, and a $1,400 smart sleeper that sensed her movements and adjusted the rocking and sound of the bed accordingly. We bought a West Elm couch and a three-foot-tall abstract painting of Buddha for the wall in the dining room. We meticulously went over the top on creating a room and home for her.

As I was getting her dressed one morning when she was four months old, I dug through her drawer full of clothes and caught the thought, *No, she wore those pants two days ago.* I laughed out loud as it occurred to me that the nursery, the clothes, were all for me. Of course I wanted her to have a beautiful, homey space to grow up in, but Pepper didn't know what pants she wore two days ago and had no idea what the hell Pottery Barn even was, let alone the ability to be grateful that her "woodland" shelf came from there.

We all want to give our kids more than we had. But we give our kids more than we had and then punish them when they're not grateful. We call them spoiled brats when they don't understand that what they have is a privilege when it's all they've ever known.

Pepper has no idea that it embarrassed me to have generic Adidas in third grade, and it won't make her appreciate the Adidas my husband will inevitably buy her when she's barely old enough to walk. (Edit: Sibe *did* end up buying her Adidas when she was three months old. She never wore them. Not once.)

What I'm starting to see is that I can't base being a good mother on giving Pepper more than I had. I can't base her appreciation, or lack thereof, on the desires and needs that I subconsciously project onto her—that she never asked for and can't understand.

What will make me a good mother to Pepper is to watch Pepper. To pay attention to *her* needs, her responses to me and her world. To notice how *she* is interpreting life and help her navigate her own path.

She doesn't need me to walk ahead of her in the jungle, torch lit, machete in hand, reaching back and saying, "Here, it's safe, I've carved the path for you." Sometimes she might. But she may also need me beside her, curious to see what's ahead and combing through dense brush together, or behind her, allowing her to stumble through it on her own.

7.

UNIVERSAL IS PERSONAL TOO

"YOU MUST BE SO EXCITED," a stranger in a coffee shop would say.

I'd half-ass an appreciative smile and choke out, "Thank you."

I wasn't excited to be pregnant. On my best day, I was devastated, trying to be accepting. And I felt completely ashamed of my feelings and smothered in guilt and afraid to tell anyone how I felt.

What if they think you don't want the baby? I would worry to myself. *Well, you don't want a baby. But that doesn't mean I don't want this one.* And *I still don't want a baby.* If there's one thing that became clear the moment I found out I was pregnant, it was that humans. Are. Complex.

I hated being pregnant. I hated the way I looked. I was embarrassed to be seen with a bump. I hated the word *bump.* I hated how people looked at me everywhere I went and always had something to say. In my case, it was even always positive, no unsolicited advice, and I still hated it. I hated how everyone I knew constantly made comments about how great I looked and my body was a constant source of conversation—that people never knew what to talk about, so they'd just always ask how I was feeling and whether or not the nursery was ready. Where had I gone? What about Vanessa the person? How about the other things that were still happening in my life outside of this human?

But mostly, I hated the assumption that I was "over the moon."

If I were over the moon the way I wanted to be, I'd be literally over the moon. I always wanted to go to space, and now I'd never be able to.

I think it's culturally irresponsible to assume that every woman experiences pregnancy from a place of excitement. The same way it's culturally irresponsible to depict birth only going the vaginal way, resulting in a tired but blissed-out mother holding her baby.

The experiences of pregnancy and motherhood are universal, but they are also deeply personal. I don't know the solution. I don't know that I would have even told a stranger how I really felt had they asked. Had I received no comments or questions, I probably would have felt badly about that too.

But I do think it's time we start to honor the incredible complexity of human emotion, especially when pregnant and into motherhood (a label that I still need to redefine for myself).

The personal and spiritual transformation that I underwent during my pregnancy is nothing short of a miracle. It's a bit like the difference between Dr. Banner and the Hulk (depending on the moment, the before or after could really be either).

I had to rearrange the universe inside of me to arrive at that point. And luckily, I had the self-awareness, coaching skill, support, and resources to do it.

I have a friend who was thrilled to be pregnant and become a mother. And she mentioned to me that while she loves it, she feels I have embraced it even more than she has. She struggles with guilt, "mom guilt," and all of the emotional convolution that comes with motherhood.

So, even her joy of pregnancy didn't translate into a purely joyful experience of motherhood. Despite the initial despair I felt, motherhood has been incredibly joyful. Two universal experiences, experienced completely personally and with many layers of emotion.

Complete selflessness can live next to frustration, guilt simultaneously with relief, commitment and exhaustion can coincide; excitement and terror, a deep knowing and resistance, can all live side by side concurrently.

It's wild. I don't think I've ever loved anything more than I love being Pepper's mother. In fact, I even love being a mother. I've enjoyed nearly every second of it in ways so profound that it surprises me daily.

I'm forever changed in the best way. Some of this is because it *is* just a *very* cool experience. The love you experience for this human blows your mind.

But I believe it would be irresponsible for me to suggest the change came about because of *becoming a mother* alone. I am changed because my pregnancy catalyzed the deepest work I'd ever done on myself. I worked for nine months with a shaman, a coach, two masterminds, and my husband and a therapist to heal deep, repressed hurt, anger, and sadness. I got incredibly honest with myself and Sibe about my judgments of mothers, my fears for our relationship, my resistance in myself, and challenged all of it. I sat in incredible discomfort, cried innumerable tears, and confronted pain that looked like it would never end, until it did.

And even after coming through "on the other side" and loving this little chicken nugget so much that it's hard to even think about anything else, there are times where I miss the sole focus that I had on work. I envy friends without this massive responsibility. I compare myself to my colleagues who are flying all over the world, taking on new and bigger contracts, being put up in five-star hotels and flying first class to get there.

I love the relaxed pace my life has now and am insanely grateful to be around Pepper so much that she probably doesn't even know

Sibe or I have a job. I love that we snuggle in bed until eight most mornings and then have breakfast and take a walk. And even as I write this, I'm typing as fast as I can because I hear her stirring from her nap, and I have to let go of the frustration trying to creep in at the limited time I have to fit work—my passion—into my life right now.

I fight for time for myself, time to work, time to work out. *And* the time I *do* have, I willingly give to Pepper.

It's complex. It's beautiful. It's frustrating, and it's catalyzing new growth.

It's calling for a bigger expansion. Work less, *and* have a bigger impact. Create time for yourself *without* giving up time with P. Experience challenges in your marriage as a result of a child, *and* become closer. Slow down your commitment to work, *and* take on bolder projects to grow your business.

In the acceptance of the complexity of the human experience, we get to expand into becoming more. That's what this journey is really all about, what it demands.

Embrace the complexity. Hold to your desires. Trust the expansion.

It's what P is asking for. It's what I want *for* her.

She's up now. And I'm *just* complete.

8.

ALL STRUCTURES ARE IMPERMANENT

FOR THE ENTIRE YEAR leading up to Pepper's birth, I struggled to access any creative energy, enthusiasm, or motivation.

For me, not only was this incredibly unusual, it was unbearably frustrating. I can't recall a time in my life where I wasn't working on something. A goal, a project, a business, growing a business, planning a trip, running a half marathon, enrolling in a course, or hiring a new coach to help me think even bigger.

For that year, though, it was like someone cut the fuel line to my creative engine.

Halfway through my partnership with my coach, I showed up to sessions saying, "Eh, I just don't really think I have anything to work on." I'd come to find later, through my work with my shaman, that this was because my spiritual evolution—catalyzed most intensely by becoming pregnant—had actually started a year before I became pregnant.

A few months after Pepper was born, it started to come back

tenfold. But the structure of my life (or lack thereof) made it tough to harness it and actually create anything. Time management felt impossible with Pepper sleeping and waking at random times. I still didn't really have the energy for follow-through. Perhaps most importantly, even though some of that creative energy was coming back online, the vast majority of my energy still just wanted to be focused on Pepper and spending time with her.

After a very frustrating Sunday when I was trying to work, watch *Gold Rush* on TV, and hang with Pepper and Sibe all at the same time, I grew increasingly agitated and decided to take Opi for a walk before I ended up bringing down Sibe's evening along with my own.

We walked around our familiar block and passed a house that I've always loved.

We live in a very hipster neighborhood that looks like it could have been pulled out of Amsterdam. But it's one of the fastest-growing neighborhoods in Pittsburgh and is mixed with countless flips and fancy new apartment buildings. New condos are popping up on every block.

I've always loved walking by this house because it's right on the main street, and it's old, poorly cared for, and has a massive yard with a fence that separates it from the sidewalk, across the street from a popular Mexican restaurant that has an incredible courtyard but overpriced, mediocre food and bewilderingly bad service. The yard was always overgrown, and there was an old container of takeout sitting on the porch on an old, white, plastic table. To me, it seemed to claim its spot defiantly against the bougie, overpriced gentrification taking place around it, and I always pictured Opi trolling the fence like a lion.

Today, this house caught my attention because it was gone.

Developers bought the property and, seemingly overnight, tore it down. All that was left was a mud lot with a fence around it. The same fence that had always been there, guarding its territory, that Opi trolled alongside in my mind hundreds of times.

The frustration and tension I had felt in my body all day drained instantly as I stood stunned, staring at the empty lot.

It was gone. This structure that had been there forever, that housed a family and a history for decades, was just gone, overnight. At first, I felt a little sad. I wondered, *If I came back to our neighborhood ten years from now, would it look like another strip mall?* Would the history and beautiful European facades be replaced with modern, glass storefronts with big brand names? Then, out of this feeling of nostalgia for a home I never lived in, something occurred to me. After a day of being so frustrated that I couldn't seem to get anything done and feeling irrelevant in the world because I wasn't able to "build" anything, it struck me that every structure is impermanent.

I was so worked up about hurrying up to rebuild my business and resurrect some kind of creative genius that I literally ruined my own day. I had forgotten that one day, whatever I feverishly built would be gone anyway.

The structure of this house that probably stood there for a hundred years was reduced to a mud lot with a fence around it in one day. The structure of my identity, of who I thought I was for thirty-three years, was reduced to confusion and internal chaos in that one moment when I looked down at a plastic stick that said, *PREGNANT.* And the business I am so focused on building—that, aside from Pepper, consumes the majority of my attention—will one day also cease to exist.

What a massive fucking relief.

I have a Zen tarot deck that uses the teachings of Osho, the mad guru from *Wild, Wild Country* who was more of a cult leader than enlightened guru. I love his teachings because they're rooted in pretty solid Zen principles, but they're peppered with just a hint of entertaining judgment and self-aggrandizement. One of my favorite cards in this deck is the "success" card. Zen teaching tells you not to get too bent out of shape about your failures, or too attached to your success. They're both fleeting. They're moments, not destinations.

Standing in this mud lot, Opi sniffing around hurriedly as if to declare that "something here is different," I saw that it almost doesn't make sense to hurry up to try to build a business at all. Or to harness all of that creative energy into building some magnificent structure. If all *structures* are impermanent, it makes more sense to focus on building moments and experiences instead.

At the very least, I certainly wouldn't want to rebuild the experiences and moments that I had created that day—half-present, fully irritated attempts at trying to be more relevant in the world, simultaneously missing everything happening around me, only misery inside of me.

There's a phrase I repeat to my clients often: "*How* you create is *what* you create." If you feel stressed in the process of building a business, your successful business will feel stressful, not satisfying. If you try to lose weight through deprivation and excessive exercise, you'll also have to maintain your lower weight through deprivation and excessive exercise. You will not feel confident and energized; you'll feel deprived and tired.

If I create a business because I'm trying to feel relevant, and stress out about not getting enough done every day, and feel half present with my family and disappointed in myself, it's unlikely that any structure I build will feel magical.

And the vision I have for my life feels like magic. The vision is not one of relevance and productivity. I dream about waking up to the ocean, taking walks on our gorgeous property, and experiencing fun and joy every moment of every day. I dream about enjoying experiences and living in the moment, but I was trying to get there by building relevant, productive structures.

I stood before this mud lot for another moment, almost to memorialize the house in my mind, and to try to integrate this realization permanently into my cells. After pulling Opi at least three times to get her to understand that we were moving again, we walked the one block back to our house.

As I reached the top of the steps, Sibe leaned forward slightly on the couch with anticipation.

"Are you feeling better?" he asked, part hopeful and part nervous.

"Yeah, I am. Thank you. Did you know they tore that house down on the corner?" I asked. "It's just a mud lot with a fence around it now."

"Huh." He shrugged, seemingly indifferent.

And I sat on the couch to finish the episode of *Gold Rush*.

9.

LATE-NIGHT LOVE

JUST AFTER GOING TO BED the other night, Pepper woke up. It was Sibe's turn, but given that I was already awake, it didn't feel right to wake him up to feed her.

She finished her bottle and snuggled up to my chest and cooed herself to sleep. I don't care how many articles tell me not to rock my babes to sleep. That's one of the most blissful, magical experiences I've ever had, and there's no way I'm going to miss out on that.

As she snuggled in closer and fell asleep, I was completely overwhelmed with love for her. My entire being melted; my breathing seemed to dissolve everything and leave just us in that perfect moment.

I watched her and saw a tiny smile cross her face. She was completely relaxed.

It felt so magical that despite my eyes trying desperately to shut from fatigue, I couldn't shut them. I had to just stare and enjoy. I didn't want to miss a second of it.

Lately, I've been trying not only to fully savor my experiences with P, but also to wonder what her experience of the very same moment is.

The more present I become in parenting, the better I'm able to remember and access feelings and memories from my own childhood that I had no idea were even there.

In this moment, I couldn't help but remember what an incredibly peaceful feeling it was to fall asleep with my mom.

That absolute loving presence felt so safe, like home.

It occurred to me how powerful this loving presence is. How, for most babies, it's the only thing they know coming into the world. To them, it *is* the world.

Specifically, my thought at that moment was *I wish I had someone to rock me to sleep like this.* And as we get older, we naturally separate from that loving presence, at least in the form of falling asleep on our parents. But we don't separate from our *need* to feel that love. I'm beginning to wonder if that's *all* we actually need to move past our personal issues and challenges within ourselves and in life.

Words from one of my clients floated into my awareness. She was talking about an insight she had while working out that week. She was being incredibly hard on herself when she paused with a sudden understanding: *You're not going to be able to hate yourself through this. You* have *to love yourself the whole way.* I imagined the thousands of times I'd beat myself up for not working out hard enough, doing enough, being productive enough, or for making a mistake.

What if I'd had my love for Pepper available to me in all of those moments?

The realization both opened my heart and made me sad in the same instance.

How powerful and immediate the shift would be, and how sad that I had denied myself that love in all of those moments.

Parenting has given me new access to that love, this time from the giver's side. I've heard that raising a baby is like a second opportunity to parent yourself.

Touching that love in that moment felt huge. So important. It's so natural, instantaneous, and automatic with her that it must just live inside me all of the time. And therefore, it exists within anyone and everyone else.

Its impact is so engulfing and so immediate.

If I can give it to her, I can give it to me.

10.
I HAVE MAGIC HANDS

I WAS LYING IN BED, trying to get Pepper to sleep after she woke up in the middle of the night. I've been trying not to pick her up every single time she cries because lately it seems to be every forty-five minutes, and I know she can't possibly be hungry again. I let her cry for a few minutes to see if she would settle back to sleep. She didn't, so I reached into her crib and found her tiny hand. She immediately grabbed my thumb and stopped crying. I lightly pinched each of her tiny chubby fingers with my index finger and thumb, going up and down each finger—a little routine we stumbled into that seems to calm her down. Back and forth a few times, and gradually her little hand went limp and I knew she'd fallen asleep. I hadn't even lifted my head off of the pillow.

I have magic hands, I think.

Being Pepper's mom is one of the coolest things in the world. For one, it is *so* awesome to be the most important person in someone's life. (Sibe may fight me on this one, rightfully. But I'm going to claim it.) I *love* being the person who can always calm her down, comfort her, and create ultimate peace. (For the record, sometimes I can't and Sibe is the one—but I'm taking this one too.)At that moment, head on the pillow, something occurred to me. As a coach, something I've become clear on over the years is that what I do, at the heart, is love my clients—even the parts of themselves that they hate, won't even acknowledge—until they love themselves. When this happens, life clicks into place, and they unleash their power to create *anything* that they want.

What if my hands could be magic everywhere? What if everyone's could?

There is a line from a song that Pepper listens to from a kundalini chant (thank you, Grandma) that says, "The sun never says to the earth 'you owe me.'"

How powerful could everyone be if we loved everyone like a mother loves her child? If we stopped keeping score of who does what, meeting the other person with complete acceptance all of the time? When Pepper is grumpy, I slow down to see what I can do to meet her needs and make her feel better. When someone we love is grumpy, it's hard not to take their mood personally or get irritated that they're bringing us down. When Pepper interrupts what I'm doing or demands all of my attention for hours, I might get tired, but I don't get resentful. I accept her fully and meet her needs as often or repetitively as they come up. I have no expectations for her, she doesn't disappoint me, and I certainly hold no judgments of what she should or shouldn't be doing.

It's an extreme idea, but I wonder what it would be like to relate to the adults in my life this way. My husband, my family and friends. The closest I come to this is with my clients. But even then, there is room for more magic.

Feeling love like this for Pepper opens up a possibility that I hadn't considered before. A possibility for so much more kindness toward other people, less judgment and more generosity. I see what it can do with Pepper. I've seen what that kind of loving presence can do with my clients over time, and it honestly is magical.

What if I had nothing but patience for my friend stuck in a toxic relationship, who wants to have the same conversation, again? What if I didn't judge myself for failing to work out for a week, and met myself with the same unconditional love no matter what my stomach looked like? What if I went in for a hug and forced a thousand kisses on Sibe's cheek when he was grumpy, and laughed when he shoved my face away with his hand like Pepper does?

A part of me, my ego, tells me that I'll be taken advantage of, rationalize my bad behavior to myself, or fail to achieve anything. But if Pepper were to try to do something that would harm her, without hesitation my loving embrace would turn into a sharp "NO." But the kind of "no" that comes from a protective love, not a judgmental attack. I could treat myself the same.

Love isn't *nice*. It's not weak, and it's anything but passive. It's honest and it's kind, but true love kills anything that isn't also love. It doesn't tolerate manipulation; it doesn't tolerate rationalization, and it's the most powerful fuel for achievement I've ever found. When we feel loved by ourselves and others, we have access to our most creative thinking, we know exactly what to do next, we see our own sabotaging patterns more clearly, and we can gain the awareness to move past them.

Love is honest in a way that says, "Turn off the TV and move your body. Get up and take time for yourself. Get to work. Take a nap. Apologize. Stand your ground." It's only in the absence of this unconditional love that we get confused about where we stand, who we are, what we should do, or how we should get there.

And you don't need to be a mother to experience this love. Being a mother just gave me more clear, constant, and direct access to this love within myself. It amplified it, but it's not different from the love I have felt thousands of times in my life before Pepper. Love always just feels like love. And nothing else feels like love. There's a particular internal quality about love that you know instantly, and you know instantly if what you're feeling is not love, though you may pretend not to know.

I've already said to Pepper a thousand times, "I'll always be here for you." And I mean it. No matter what she does or what unfolds in our life or between us, I will always be there for her. I'll always love her, waiting patiently and steadily.

A coach of mine used to say, "The path is always there waiting for you. It doesn't judge you when you step off, no matter how long. It doesn't get upset with you for standing still on it when you should be moving. It doesn't waver, it doesn't change. It just waits for you to get back on when you're ready."

That's the kind of love I'm talking about. That's what having magic hands really means. It's the kind of love I feel for Pepper all of the time and the kind of love that has always been present in me, and is present in everyone. The more you practice connecting to it, the harder it is to disconnect from it.

That's when the real magic begins.

11.

NOT MORE *LOVE*; FEWER CONDITIONS

LOVING PEPPER IS TEACHING ME to love everyone else more, especially Sibe.

For one, I love her so much it makes my heart want to explode. My capacity to feel love pushes constantly up against its edges, feeling like fear but actually voicing a constant request for my heart to expand to hold more love.

As I acknowledge this new capacity, it shines a light on where I can expand the love I have for others—in this case, Sibe.

It's not that I love Pepper more than Sibe. But I definitely love her with fewer conditions. I love everything Pepper does. Every cry, every poop, every frustrated episode, exploration, discovery, smile, and evolution. I marvel at every tiny evolution in skill, development, and personality.

I'm conscious of asking "Who are you?" moment to moment with curiosity to let her show me, instead of projecting a personality onto her. ("Pepper. She must be spicy, right?") And when she does show me an aspect of herself, I'm careful not to box her into that display so that she can be whomever she wants at any moment. And love all of it.

Juxtaposed against this, I became aware of how many conditions I put on my love for Sibe. How easily triggered I am, how much I mentally force him to be what I want him to be rather than who he is (and how much he does this to me).

I want him to care less about details I think are stupid, I want him to like our dog more, I want him to stress less about some things and care more about others. I want him to like sitting in coffee shops with me, to enjoy lingering after the check is paid at a restaurant, to feel differently about people in general.

I decide who he is and react to those decisions. I decide that he judges me and therefore receive loving comments as judgments. I decide how he'll respond before I even ask him things. I paint the caricature of him in my mind and then expect and project it onto him before he even has a chance to show me something else. And when he does, I distort that reality to match my image of him. We all do this.

But I love Pepper exactly as she is. No conditions. I meet all of my experiences of her with wonder, curiosity, compassion, and delight. Aside from a few instances, even when she deprives me of sleep for months on end, I can't wait for her to wake up crying at 3 a.m. to eat.

I literally complain to Sibe regularly about him waking me up from a nap by talking too loudly on the phone.

At first, my massive Pepper love scared me. It felt like it dwarfed and overshadowed all of the other love in my life. I thought it meant that I loved Pepper more than Sibe and that eventually this would drive a wedge between us and he would become my co-parent or, worse, errand boy.

Part of this was conditioning around what happens to your marriage when you have children. But part of it is what I believe to be "growing pains" of the heart.

Our experiences can be simplified into fear-based or love-based.

In other words, you're either feeling fear or love. That's it.

When our capacity to love expands, it pushes up against and crowds out fear. The growing love pushes the boundaries of your heart. You've never felt this much love before, so it feels like you can only push so far before it ends, triggering fear and worry.

Not because the love will actually run out, or overshadow. Simply because fear is vying for its spot.

When I experience this massive love for Pepper, fear tells me I love her *more* than Sibe, that it casts a shadow. When I look at this from love, it shows me the extra capacity I have to love Sibe. It shines a light on the space available.

What if I loved Sibe like I loved Pepper, exactly as he is? No conditions. What if I met all of my experiences of him with wonder, curiosity, compassion, and delight? Even when he deprives me of sleep for months on end. What if I couldn't wait for him to wake me up from a nap by talking too loudly on the phone?

In Zen teaching, they explain that most people don't experience true love. They experience neediness in disguise. They need the other person in order to feel whole; they need the other person to change to fit their mold so they can feel "love."

But true love is not conditional. True love asks you to be endlessly open to allowing others to shine light on the places where you're triggered and heal them in yourself to meet their triggers with love. It asks you to not ask anything of them and to love them as they are. It asks for your wholeness to meet their wholeness.

So, I'm seeing this differently. Not all the time—not even close to as much as I'd like to.

Maybe love is like matter. It can't be created or destroyed. It can only be distorted through the conditions we place on it.

Being Pepper's mom has allowed me to experience love without conditions, and it blows me away.

A book called *The Couple's Tao Te Ching* shares how to apply the ancient wisdom to all love and relationships.

In it, it shares the following:

Love dances through the cosmos,
binding together all that is.
Every living thing is welcomed
with never a word of criticism.
Welcome each other
with the same expansiveness.
What pleases you
and does not please you
is of no importance.
Welcome is all that matters.

12.

I NEED COMPASSION AND I'LL RAGE UNTIL I GET IT

"WANT TO REFILL MY COFFEE?" Sibe asked me cheerily as I stomped past him and Pepper playing on the couch one morning.

"No." I walked by, staring straight ahead.

"That was a grumpy no!" he replied, with amused surprise.

Cue Metallica and the subtle scent of burning cars.

We had just started sleep training with P, and instead of sleeping in until nine with her like I usually did, we got up at seven so we could get her on a different schedule. Since we made the agreement that I would do the night feedings, I felt like I was the only one bearing the weight of the new change. I was incredibly tired, and indeed very grumpy. Was that Sibe's fault? No. Did he know any of this was going on? Absolutely not.

I knew what I needed to do: tell him that I was insanely tired from this new change. That what I really needed was for him to make me a cup of tea, give me a hug and a kiss on the forehead, and tell me we'd get through this new phase together and to go take a shower while he played with Pepper.

My higher self: *I know what I need to do.*

My not higher self: *Hold my beer.*

Sibe: "You seem grumpy," he repeated as he and Pepper cheerily bounced into the room where I was obviously pouting on the bed. "Pepper, your mom is grumpy!"

Not-higher-self Vanessa: "*Grumpy? GRUMPY?* Instead of calling me grumpy, how about coming in here and offering to make me tea? Seeing that I'm tired and giving me a kiss on the forehead and actually noticing what I need?"

Higher-self Vanessa: Facepalm.

Perhaps obviously to everyone else, this did not work to effectively elicit the compassionate response I was hoping for.

Instead, higher-self Sibe responded, "Stop it, Vanessa." (I hate when he says that. Immediately I know he's right.) "We both know I'm always supportive, and if you need help, ask for it. Don't do this. Go take a nap."

With that, he and Pepper bounced back out of the room.

I lay back down with adrenaline pumping through my veins. I put a T-shirt over my eyes and tried to take a rage nap. I thought of storming into the living room to reiterate my point. I even thought about squirting him with the water bottle we use to clean off Pepper's butt.

Higher-self Vanessa: *Let it go.*

I made an agreement with myself years ago that the moment I am sure I'm right, I drop it. This assurance that I'm right paired with a feeling of spastic frustration is a clear sign that I'm acting like an idiot. A tired idiot, but an idiot nonetheless. 100 percent of the time. Also 100 percent of the time, I believe that this is the time that I am *actually* right.

A kinder way to explain what was happening, and what we all do in varying degrees, is that I was acting like Pepper. I was asking for love like an infant.

When Pepper needs something, she loses her shit. That's what babies do. They cry and escalate until you finally guess what's wrong and lovingly and patiently meet the need and calm the tears with a loving embrace. Moreover, you anticipate their needs in order to avoid babies losing their shit in the first place. That's what mommies and daddies do.

It's not what adult human beings in adult relationships do.

Unless they're tired or "not-higher-self Vanessa." Tired, adult, not-higher-self Vanessa doesn't get love and affection when she wraps herself in barbed wire, plants landmines around herself, and then runs into the room screaming, "SOMEONE GIVE ME A HUG, GODDAMNNIT!"

When she does that, people run away. And then she blames them for not supporting her.

We all do this. We are only somewhat conscious of our own needs. We're more aware of the discomfort and frustration of our unmet needs. It's more obvious to us when other people don't give us what we have not yet asked for—what we have not even acknowledged to ourselves that we need.

And then we punish them before we've given them a chance to meet those requests that we have not yet made.

I've coached just about every client I've ever worked with on this very topic and offered them this strategy:

Create a greater awareness of your needs.

Acknowledge *and accept* the needs you have.

Communicate those needs to the people around you.

Don't assume they will know them or see them.

Receive the meeting of those needs.

Repeat when they forget.

Thank them when they remember.

And yet, as most do, I continually forget this when I'm in moments of lower consciousness.

Later that day, I apologized, to which Sibe replied that he had let it go hours ago and didn't take it personally in the first place.

He also suggested that it was time to revisit how we handle P's feeding, since the schedule was changing and it no longer made sense for me to do the full night alone.

This is a lesson that I continue to both learn and teach.

As an infant, it makes perfect sense for Pepper to expect me to anticipate her needs and patiently try different things when she's crying for something. When we carry that same behavior into our adult relationships, it creates unnecessary expectations, disappointment, and resentment.

Once we grow up, it's our responsibility to understand and acknowledge our own needs and communicate them *with* love, to receive love.

In summary: stop asking for love like an infant.

13.

WHY NOT JUST ENJOY IT?

THIS STORY IS PROBABLY going to let a little too much of my crazy show.

A few months after P was born, I was having dinner at the house of a friend who had a baby just a few weeks before me. We were talking about sleep schedules, and she mentioned how she follows a principle called "sleep, eat, play."

She kept mixing the salad and checking the baby monitor. "That's what we do all day: sleep, eat, play—in that order."

"What do you do to play?" I asked.

"Anything. Tummy time, his play mat, walk around and listen to music."

"How long do you do each thing?" *God, Vanessa, shut up.* I could hear how insane I was sounding. I also made a mental note that walking around listening to music counted as playing.

"He lets me know when he's done."

I thought about it the entire next day. *Okay. Got it. Sleep, eat, play. Simple enough.* Pepper woke up from her nap. *Sleep, check.* I fed her. *Yep. Got this. Playtime.*

I stared at P. Nothin'. *What am I supposed to do with a three-month-old? I guess it has to do with development at this point. What needs to be developed?*

I remembered I had an app for this! It told me what activities to do at each age of development.

I laid P down on the couch and whipped it out.

"Select five of the nine activities." Easy enough.

I was met with options like "head lift, reach for toy, hold the bottle, narrate your actions." I kid you not, the next thought in my head was *Which one of these is the easiest?* Followed by *How long are you supposed to have her reach for the toy? Or is this measured in reps?* This went on until I reached the option "bond with your baby." And the instructions were to lie down, make eye contact, snuggle her, and basically bond with your fucking baby.

What the hell is wrong with me?

Opi banged on the bell to go outside.

I was desperate for a break, and Sibe wouldn't be home for another hour. I felt a little restless; my mind was racing, as if the faster it worked, the more I could outthink this uncomfortable feeling. Given that I was trapped for at least another hour and it was a gorgeous fall night, I decided to take the monsters (myself included) for an evening walk.

I just couldn't shake the feeling that I should be doing something, couldn't help wondering if I had done enough or if I was doing everything right. The words of my aunt (who happens to be a midwife) popped into my head: "Here's a thought. Why don't you just *enjoy* your baby?" she teased me. I had her on speed dial from day one, asking her hurried, stressed-out questions like "How long do I breastfeed on each side? What if she falls asleep while she's eating? She hates tummy time; what should I do? Should I time her? I read online that she should be doing an hour a day by month three. She won't even do ten seconds." And I would know, because I literally used a stopwatch to time tummy time.

When she heard that we were clocking tummy time with a stopwatch and using an app that tracked how long Pepper breastfed on each side, she just about lost it laughing, genuinely concerned that I had lost my mind.

Just enjoy it, I thought again. Honestly, I had never considered that. It felt like everything was too high stakes. Nowhere online did I read, *Why don't you just enjoy it?* when I Google-searched *How long should a four-week-old breastfeed?* But it was freeing. It reminded me that women have been having babies as long as there have been women—when apps didn't exist, and neither did stopwatches.

I relaxed a little. I laughed to myself, thinking about more primal women counting to track breastfeeding time, etching a tally on the wall under the cave drawing of a left boob. I looked down at P sleeping in the stroller and Opi sniffing along the edge of the sidewalk, both enjoying themselves.

My energy shifted from restless, counting down the minutes until Sibe came home, to a slower, more present awareness of my surroundings. I became aware of just how nice the evening was. Yes, I was tired, but in a sleepy, slow way that almost matched the speed of the early-fall dusk evening. My hands relaxed their grip on the stroller slightly, and I felt some of the tension leave my body when Opi wanted to stop for the four hundredth time to sniff a tree.

14.

I DIDN'T EXPECT THIS

WE WERE ON VACATION in Florida with Sibe's family when I sat down with my mother-in-law to share, honestly, how hard for me the first eight weeks of Pepper's life had been, including her visit. I was afraid to share this with her, but my fear of repeating those first weeks gave me anxiety. I hadn't really known how to communicate what I needed and was reminded by Sibe that if I didn't communicate anything, no one would know anything was happening. I didn't want to hurt her feelings, or offend anyone, but I really wanted to enjoy my trip.

When I shared all of this with her, I was met with nothing but love. Her main concern was that I hadn't felt secure enough to tell her what I needed or that she somehow made it seem like I couldn't share what had been happening for me during her previous visit. She shared some of the experiences that were hard for her, and I held space for that too. I confessed that, perhaps irrationally, if Pepper cried, I wanted to be the one to care for her. Despite knowing that anyone else was capable, I wanted it to be me. It was too hard to hear her cry, be in the room, and have someone else handling it. She agreed without hesitation and with complete empathy.

When I shared my difficulties with my sisters, their main concern was that they hoped that they didn't contribute to that struggle and asked how they could help me more. Unsurprisingly, I was not met with judgment of being a jerk, irrational, or selfish.

Later that day, P started crying, and without skipping a beat, my mother-in-law grabbed her from my brother-in-law, handed her to me, and winked.

All of a sudden, I had an ally.

It felt like such a relief, and at the same time, it was surprisingly difficult. Once I had Pepper back, I started to question my own needs. *Am I being ridiculous? Why shouldn't I leave her with them while I nap? Let someone else take care of her.* I discovered that I was actually the one stealing P from myself in those first eight weeks. Each time I handed her away when I didn't want to, but didn't communicate it, I was stealing her from me. I was the one having a hard time honoring my own needs, which is why I couldn't communicate them and others could not meet them.

In that space, I discovered my newest challenge was to receive the love and support I asked for. When I started this journey, my goal was to expand my capacity to love. To love everyone around me—my baby, my family, my clients, and my husband—more.

I wanted to see how this impacted my ability to enjoy, create, and earn.

I didn't expect that a part of expanding my ability to give love would also challenge me to expand my ability to receive love.

It reminded me of a story I read in *Messages from the Masters*, about the lessons we have to learn in each of our lives, by Brian Weiss. The story was about a mother, an older woman who had several adult children. One day, her daughter, a doctor, came to visit. Out of the blue, she said to her daughter, "If anything ever happened to me, where I wasn't able to care for myself, promise me that you'll end my life. Only you have the ability to do this for me." Her daughter laughed it off, though slightly disturbed by the request. A short time later, her mother had a stroke, leaving her mental faculties in perfect condition but her body paralyzed. The daughter remembered the request, but couldn't bring herself to follow through with it. After four years, her mother died.

In a meditation one day, the daughter heard a voice.

"Why are you so angry with me?" God asked.

Furious, the daughter replied, "Because my mother didn't deserve that. All she ever did was take care of other people for her entire life. She gave and gave selflessly and she deserved more than that punishment."

"What I did for your mother was mercy," God replied.

"MERCY?!" she demanded. "How was that torture mercy? She was a proud woman. To live the last four years of her life like that was dehumanizing and terrible for her."

"Your mother *only* gave," God replied lovingly. "She spent her entire life giving and never receiving. The cycle of giving must be balanced with receiving so that others may also give. What your mother learned in four years at the end of her life may have taken her many more lifetimes to learn in much more difficult ways had I not intervened. Through this experience, she was required to receive constant love, support and care from others. However painful it may have been for her ego, her soul learned the value of receiving. She learned this very important lesson in a very short time."

The story struck me profoundly—in part because a good threat can go a long way with me when I'm being hard-headed: "Receive now or pay later." But mainly because I had not really thought about this before.

In my business I had. In order for me to generate income, I serve people. I give so that I can receive. And I have coached many clients to this same understanding. They struggled to earn money, continuing to invest in more and more training to become more qualified, but failed to really help people, to give—requirement to receive. I was clear on how the cycle worked.

I just hadn't considered it in my personal life.

But this simple gesture from my mother-in-law, taking Pepper from my brother-in-law and handing her to me, and the discomfort that it created in me, woke me up in a subtle way that I'm sure I will need to wake up a thousand more times before I really wake up to it.

I've been on a journey to expand my capacity to love. "To love," like a verb, a thing I'm doing. But I can see now that if I'm going to expand my capacity to give love, then I will also have to expand my capacity to tolerate love. One meaning of the word *tolerate* is "to allow without interference."

For it to flow, it has to be both given and received. To give love better, one must allow more love back, without interference.

15.

BOUNDARIES

I ONCE HELD PEPPER for two hours on a flight. When I deboarded the plane, I carried her off as she slept and waited for Sibe while he grabbed our luggage. It took about ten or so minutes before he arrived with the stroller.

It wasn't until I put her down that I realized how much pain my arm was in—that feeling when your elbow has been bent for so long that when you finally extend it, it's almost impossible to move.

That's kind of what motherhood is like. It's not that you intentionally neglect your own needs; you're just so tuned in to the needs of your nugget and your responsibilities that, likely a strategy of evolution, you don't even notice that your arm feels like it's about to fall off until you put her down.

Just before I had Pepper, tons of people shared the importance of setting boundaries, both with visitors and in terms of taking time for yourself. I failed to do this.

I failed to communicate my true needs when we had visitors and I needed space, or wanted Pepper back. I failed to communicate that

I was having a hard time. I failed to ask for the help I needed in the way I needed it. I failed to communicate that the help that was being offered was not the help I wanted. I failed to take time or space for myself.

I spent months thinking about how this happened. I thought I would want a full-time nanny. I thought I would want someone to hold my baby. I thought I would want time alone. As someone who never has an issue sharing honestly with the people I love, I thought I wouldn't have any issues communicating my needs. I thought I would recognize my needs. I thought I would have the courage to speak them when I did.

After contemplating and exploring this for months, this is what I discovered. I failed in all of these things because there is a prerequisite to setting boundaries. Before you can effectively set boundaries, you first have to understand your needs. You can't set a boundary when you don't even know the line. And this experience was so new, so unfamiliar, so primal, and it conflicted so much with how I *thought* I would feel that I was in a constant state of confusion and didn't even know it. My normal guidance system completely fell off-line.

I had no idea how much I had been affected by the delivery. It wasn't until nearly three months after Pepper's birth that I acknowledged how deeply, deeply hurt I was that I was unconscious through it and how angry I was that I felt something had been stolen from me.

I had no idea I was recreating that experience every time I handed Pepper to someone and didn't want to. I didn't realize that I was trying to constantly make up for that feeling of lack by trying to steal more and more time with her in the present. I had an almost compulsive need to be with her to try to steal back some of the time I felt I had lost, a totally unworkable equation.

I didn't even really know what my body was going through. I didn't know the extent to which primal instincts kick in and how painful it would be to hear my baby cry. I didn't know how impatient

I would feel when anyone other than me tried to tend to her. And I didn't know it was okay for me to just tell the people I loved that if she cried, I wanted to tend to her, no questions asked.

I didn't know it was okay to do all of that. I judged it as selfish. I judged my needs as irrational. I judged my desire to hold Pepper even while our families were in town as selfish because they lived so faraway. I judged my need for space as rude, so I didn't ask for it. I couldn't see what I needed in the moment because I was so overly concerned with trying to help create a beautiful experience for others that I was torturing myself. And then I would notice a pang of something inside and dismiss it as quickly as it came, never even pausing to check in with what I was asking myself for.

The result was intense anger, a pattern I've been working to shift. On the surface, it really looked like I was angry at everyone else. How did they not see my needs? Why didn't they care more about *me* than the baby?

The better question was, how did *I* not see my needs? Why didn't I care more about me than everyone around me?

It was too easy for me to stay mad at my family for not tending to my needs. It was too hard to admit that I had done such a good job denying my needs that they didn't stand a chance at seeing them. It wasn't until *weeks* later that I even noticed that I had them and that they weren't met.

In the end, I was angry at myself. It was my job to set boundaries.

Something else I see now, though, is that boundaries aren't even necessary when you understand your needs. I wouldn't have had to set boundaries with my family. I discovered this when I had that conversation with my mother-in-law on vacation. She didn't ridicule me for my primal desires. In fact, she repeatedly saved me from crossing my *own* boundaries and helped me to enforce them with others. There's no doubt in my mind that every single other family member who visited in that time would have done the same.

So, the fault is mine.

But "fault" only lies as deep as your consciousness or awareness in any moment goes. You can only choose from the options you see in any moment, and your ability to see, *really* see, is more complex than just doing what you "know" to be right.

Often, when I am with Sibe in the Netherlands, where he is from, my brain gets fatigued from practicing and listening to Dutch for days, something it's not accustomed to and which is still quite challenging for me. After a few days, I don't even hear it anymore. I might be sitting at a table and Sibe will say, "Do you understand what we're talking about?" Occasionally the honest answer is "I actually didn't even *hear* any talking."

The brain is so good at filtering foreign sounds as a way of helping you not be overwhelmed by your environment that it can tune out sounds you *do* need to hear. Of course, you need this protection so that you can focus on what is important. In my day-to-day, Dutch would be an erroneous noise distracting me from speaking and thinking in English. But when the context of my environment changes and I am in Holland, Dutch becomes a very important sound. My brain simply hasn't caught up and continues to "help me" by filtering it out.

Consciousness and awareness work similarly. We get really good at filtering the internal noise to best suit us to our world. From a very young age, we start to set conditions for which internal experiences help us and which ones make life harder. This becomes so patterned, it happens on its own. Unconsciously. Without your awareness.

If awareness shows up at all, as my needs did in those early weeks, it competes with other needs that have a higher spot in your consciousness, so you register that awareness as dissonance, confusion, or a perceived threat to the balance of your environment. So, subconsciously, with limited awareness, you push them aside.

In other words, without your full permission, your brain creates a hierarchy of needs and then matches them up to the environment and then, based on your current experiences, filters the needs that arise against the hierarchy it's created, and you have very little say in this process.

We mostly only become aware that this process is happening when the pain of the sorting becomes great enough to notice. I suppose I just happen to have a high threshold for pain. Useful in some circumstances—not as useful when I accumulate so much pain that I want to erupt like a volcano, and then it comes out as anger and frustration toward others. This is all embarrassing to admit. Childish and immature, it's a strategy I took on as a kid; it worked then, and I just never upgraded it until now. And even now, these upgrades take time.

Yet, even with all of this internal noise, your needs are there, asking to be heard.

A tiny triangle amid the big brass band. Always audible if you've learned to pay attention to how it shows up. My big brass band shows up as being annoyed, frustrated, martyred, and rageful. Tension in my chest, anxiety in my body, a desperate fear of running out of time, and a need to tell people off.

My triangle is a sensation in my gut and heart. Barely noticeable, easy to miss, followed by an even easier-to-dismiss feeling that occurs just *after* I ignore a need—much easier to ignore than the rush of frustration in my chest, especially when set against the fear of upsetting someone or a desire to create a great experience for someone else.

But this subtle sensation is where your boundaries are born; it's your body making requests, your needs coming to the surface.

I've discovered that it is both my job and my *practice* to listen more closely, past the sound of heavy horns and percussion, for the tiny chime patiently ringing behind it all.

16.

THERE'S NEVER ENOUGH TIME

THERE'S NEVER ENOUGH TIME when you're ahead of life, out of integrity, or out of your mind.

I was rocking Pepper to sleep, finally feeling calm for the first time in about twelve hours, when this occurred to me.

The last twenty-four hours had been incredibly stressful. No matter how I seemed to organize my time, something always came up to disrupt the plan I'd set. Despite most of those things being of my own doing, I felt completely overwhelmed, disempowered, and frustrated.

I was running through the list of things I, for the millionth time this month, hadn't gotten done, or even started. Over the past few days, I kept repeating the phrase, "I just do not have enough time." I have a tendency to always be ahead of life. Starting our new business, I already want it to be so much more successful than it's ready to be. It's a brand-new business, and I resent our lack of progress when I sit down to work on it. The frustration that builds as a result makes it impossible to focus and even more impossible to connect to my intuition and clarity to be able to see what step makes sense to take next. Despite knowing exactly what to do in my coaching business and being able to help my clients with this challenge all the time, I myself get completely paralyzed when I work on this business.

Because I want it to be where it's not yet ready to be, I am ahead of life. In the make-believe reality I am living in, there aren't steps to take. I'm looking for a result that would come from action I haven't taken. No matter how much more time I have to work, it will never feel like enough if I don't slow down internally and allow my progress to be what it is in *this* moment. Only then can I see the next step. My coach once shared with me, "You can't see the next step because you haven't taken the one in front of you yet. So, you're not supposed to be able to see it."

The reality is that while I have control over my actions, I have very little control over the way and the timeline with which results unfold. When I forget this and try to control results instead of my actions, life gets very, very hard, and it only *looks* like more time is the solution.

As for the integrity part, I have a lot going on, and I support a lot of people. Between my kid, my dog, myself, my husband, and my clients, I have a lot of commitments. The truth is that I have plenty of time to meet these commitments. But when I let my integrity slip—when I spend ten minutes on social media that turns into thirty, or sit down to write but end up writing an email to my clients, or talk to my sister for an hour when she picks up Pepper, or even run over twenty minutes on a call with a client—it's easy to forget that I have enough time.

Being out of integrity simply means you are not doing what you said you would be doing.

When I arrange the work I want to do each day, I do it based on what I'd like to accomplish in the time I have available. But without integrity, the day ends and I find myself frustrated because I didn't complete half of what I wanted to get done. I panic about not having enough time.

More time won't help where there is a lack of integrity. What I didn't see until this moment, rocking Pepper to sleep, was that more time can only help when you use that time effectively. So even when I did manage to find more time, or get more help, I still ended up not getting done what I needed to because I didn't have enough integrity in the time I had.

So, let's say you're on pace with life and you're in integrity with what you say you want to do. More time still won't help when you're out of your mind. By that I mean, for example, trying to rebuild your business, build a new business, write two books, and raise your first baby with fifteen hours of childcare a week. Sometimes I am just simply out of my mind when I take on what I take on in the first place. It's a habit I used to try to break. Upon realizing that it appears to be wired into my DNA, I relax, knowing that more time will probably only make the issue worse. More time will likely present another idea that I'll happily take on, adding more to my already impossible list. The solution, then, when you're out of your mind, is a longer time *horizon*. If I'm not willing to take anything off my plate, then I simply need to acknowledge that I'll be finishing this meal at a much later date than anticipated.

"There's never enough time when you're ahead of life, out of integrity, or out of your mind."

17.

THE WORK YOU NEED TO DO

EVERYONE HAS INNER WORK they need to do and inner work they want to do—the growth they need, and the growth they think they need. The growth I thought I needed was to make endless amounts of money and reach ever-higher levels of success. The growth I really needed was to learn how to be present and feel safe in my life. For most of my life, standing still—literally and metaphorically—sent torrents of anxious energy through my body. And that energy would fuel me. I would work twelve hours straight with no lunch because pausing for fifteen minutes made me feel like I was falling behind.

The physical manifestation of this was a perfect mirror image. I had three consecutive months where I earned $45K, $55K and $35K. And each of those months, I overdrew my bank account.

Let me repeat that. I earned $45K in a month and *spent* more. I earned $55K in a month and *spent* more the following month. And then I earned $35K in a month and spent more.

I earned $135K in three months and netted *negative* one hundred dollars from paying overdraft fees.

I was a bottomless pit for and of money and success. All of the inner work I did was really only to elevate myself professionally and financially. I would have denied that to death if you had asked me. But that's how good we can be at deceiving ourselves.

And I always had more work to do because I was solving the wrong problem.

The work I needed to do was on how I processed traumatic childhood events, completely repressed sadness for any reason, past or present, and channeled it into anger and drive, and then wondered why I felt like I constantly had a ghost chasing me that I couldn't outrun. Or should I say, out-earn or achieve. I needed to learn how to process stress, anger, change, and difficult emotions—and perhaps, above all, to be vulnerable, open my heart to others, and receive love and support.

We all have our lie. "More success and money are the answer" was mine.

It's like having a goal to swim across the Chesapeake Bay and only training to do it by running marathons. It *almost* makes sense. You worked really hard, you trained your cardiovascular endurance, and you're in great health. But you get in the water and nearly drown because you didn't practice swimming. So you tell yourself you just need to run a little more to get your lung capacity up a little higher. You need to start swimming.

My goal was to feel happy and content with my life. So I would work, achieve, and feel relief. Momentarily (and I literally mean a moment), I would feel safe, secure, successful. But a moment later, it would dissipate, and my chest would light up with that familiar anxious feeling. The old alarm bells would ring. I would tell myself that I just needed a little more success, a little more money. It kind of made sense. But I was running, not swimming.

Had I not gotten pregnant, I really doubt that I would have ever done that work. I believed my lie too much. And I was too good at making it work (if by making it work you mean earning a shit ton of money but spending it before you can use it, sinking further into debt and confusion). I knew in my heart that if I ever wanted kids, I'd have to do that work, but I was never going to want kids until I did that work. The perfect escape to remain "not a mother." But the anguish that erupted when I got pregnant was too much to ignore.

I was drowning, and the faster I tried to run, the deeper I sank.

The anxiety that kept me running my entire life didn't even bother to show up. It was like, on a completely unconscious level, I knew that money and success couldn't solve this.

That year before I got pregnant, when I had trouble being creative, I kept saying, "It feels like someone cut my fuel line to my creativity. I keep pressing on the gas, but I'm not really moving anymore."

It didn't make any logical sense. But I've started to pay attention to those completely illogical but persistent experiences that happen on a soul and cellular level.

It was time to do the work I needed to do.

I let myself drown. I let myself sink through the guilt and shame for feeling this way about this unborn human. In reality, I wasn't even thinking about her. I was thinking about me. And I had to let myself drown and sink into grief, fear, and sadness to see that what I actually craved was relief from the person I had become. I was exhausted. I was desperately attached to controlling every outcome in my life, and desperately tired of being me. And at the same time, desperately afraid not to be.

I had no idea that I was being given a gift. An opportunity to, however reluctantly, let go of a way of being and a strategy for living that only kind of worked and begin to access a new depth of experience.

I find it so important to reiterate that motherhood in and of itself didn't magically make me into a fulfilled and happy human being, and Pepper alone didn't make me love being her mother. I'm sure I would have loved her as much without doing this work, but my sense is that it would have been a complete mess of complex, constantly conflicting energy and emotion. "I love you, but I resent you." Do we even dare say that out loud? Because I bet my house that there are thousands of mothers walking around tortured by that unspoken experience. But living life from this perspective allows all of your pain to teach you where to go next to evolve.

For me, in that moment, the pain was motherhood. Which meant my access point to my own evolution was motherhood, the most profound opportunity yet. Later in life, it might be a career opportunity, a professional failure, or the loss of something or someone I love.

One of my favorite spiritual teachings is about a woman who asks her teacher, "I keep having a nightmare. It's terrifying. I am running down a hallway and there are monsters chasing me. I know that if they find me, they'll kill me, and I can feel their breath on the back of my hair as they get closer. I know they're going to catch me, and just before they do, I wake up."

"What do the monsters look like?" her teacher asks.

"I have no idea; I'm always running with them behind me. It's terrifying. When I wake up, I'm exhausted as if I've actually been running, and I can't fall back to sleep. It stays with me for days."

"Next time you have the dream, turn around and look at them."

"But they'll kill me!"

"Then let them."

She agrees to turn around the next time she has the dream.

The next time, she's running down the hallway, feeling their breath on the back of her head, when she remembers her commitment to turn around to look at them. Terrified, she turns.

She shares with her teacher, "I almost couldn't bring myself to do it. I was so certain that they would kill me. But when I turned around, something incredible happened. They kept running at me, and then, like there was some invisible force field, they couldn't get any closer. They just stood there thrashing around, not able to get any closer. At first I found them horrifying. Terrible, thrashing, and ugly. But after

I stood there for a while, they became pathetic, and then I even felt a bit sorry for them. And in that moment, they disappeared."

My monsters were rage, anger, sadness, abandonment, fear, and loneliness. I was angry at my own mother for the mistakes she made when I was a kid. I felt rage toward my father for who he was, who I saw him as, and for not being able to share or work through that anger as a kid. And I was angry at God for abandoning me.

I developed a strategy of repressing everything hard and channeling it into drive. On a subconscious level, I believed that if I repressed those feelings and could just become successful enough, I would feel connected and loved, and a sense of community. But each time I repressed a difficult emotional experience, I felt disconnected, and this created an incredible sense of loneliness in life. Until I was thirty-three years old, I was terrified of life. People always told me how brave I was. Inside I would say, *I'm not brave because I want to be; I'm brave because I have to be.* I was terrified of the unknown, I didn't trust life, and I felt that *everything* was on my shoulders.

It was like I had constructed a perfectly built city—a million tiny details carefully pieced together to construct a place unlike any other, vast and almost overwhelming in its size and complexity. To the outside world, impressive, expansive, and powerful. Only it was built out of cards, and a strong enough breeze would bring the entire thing to the ground.

Getting pregnant was a gale-force wind, and I knew it was going to take my entire city down.

I still don't quite know why. Maybe something about being self-reliant, and now I had to take care of another human. Maybe because the only thing I had ever truly valued was success and drive, and I couldn't afford to have another priority. Success was life and death.

And this new life meant my death.

At least, death to my way of seeing the world and of seeing myself. And while it was the death of a false me, the ego—like all living things—fights to survive and fears its own death.

The ego knows nothing of being but thinks it can save itself through doing. I knew on a deep level that *being* a mother meant I could no longer be *doing* life the way I had before.

In the car on the way home after our ultrasound that confirmed our pregnancy was viable, Sibe asked me, "I feel like we have to at least ask this. Do we want to go through with this? Do *you* want to go through with this? We don't have to."

But we did have to. Not from some moral standpoint about abortion; there just didn't seem to be any choice to make.

It was my soul who cut the fuel line to my motivation and drive to work endlessly on my business a year before; it was also my soul who, when I discovered I was pregnant, quietly sat, statuesque in her assuredness, rooted entirely in her confidence, and said, "Yes. We're doing this."

18.
MISUNDERSTOOD

I HAD A CLIENT YEARS AGO who struggled with a deep, deep sense of being unlovable.

We probably coached on this topic dozens of times in the year that we worked together. Each time, I tried to support her to move through it to create a different experience, but she seemed to become more and more frustrated with me. I didn't understand her pain, and therefore she felt deeply misunderstood by me.

In complete transparency, I was frustrated by this and on some level must have thought that she wanted to hold on to her pain.

To this person: I am so sorry. You *were* deeply misunderstood.

Only now, three months into motherhood and more than two years after working with her, do I understand what it really means to feel so misunderstood.

What I think she was trying to say was that no matter how much I could see where she was coming from in my head, I couldn't possibly feel the pain that was in her heart. And until I could completely understand that, there was no way I could understand her. I couldn't understand why the little things that shouldn't have upset her so much did. How seemingly small incidences felt like assaults to her heart. How no matter how much she tried to explain it, she always sounded crazy out loud, and how disappointing it was to explain how she felt as best she could, only to see on the face of whoever was listening that they still didn't get it.

I get it now.

The first few months of Pepper's life were intense.

I felt angry about the birth, angry at my body. I was grieving having missed the birth and didn't know it, and, on top of it, I was exhausted from hosting out-of-town guests.

I was so happy for Pepper to spend time with her family and our friends, and so determined to be a gracious host, that I completely suppressed and ignored the constant pull of my intuitive impulse to create space and quiet to bond with this new little human.

And it killed me inside. One small instance at a time, these little assaults to my intuition accumulated, and I completely broke down.

For months after, I felt like I couldn't get close enough to Pepper. I was on the verge of tears all the time and didn't understand why. I felt intense anger that I later learned was repressed sadness from feeling so separated from her in those first eight weeks and from everything that had transpired in her delivery.

And when I finally did try to share it, I felt deeply misunderstood.

I can totally understand why. I could hear and feel the intense anger and energy in my voice that didn't match the scenario I was explaining.

How could it feel so hard to have people you love surrounding you, loving your baby, cleaning your house, cooking for you, buying you gifts, and going out for meals and fun outings?

They would say things like, "I get it. Your hormones are all over the place and this is new for you. You're doing a great job."

These words would upset me even more. I was only doing a great job hiding the fact that I was on the edge of a complete breakdown.

I was furious for feeling like I had to do a great job doing something that felt terrible to do.

I didn't have the self-awareness to communicate what I wanted. That what I really need is to hold my baby as much as I want, to take her from them when she cries even though I know they can just as easily meet her needs. That, as much as I love them, I need them to give me space, lots of space—and then come back when I need them. And to spend time with the baby by sitting next to me as *I* hold her. And to not receive my edginess as being hormonal or irrational. To not see my need to take care of my crying baby as interfering. To pay attention to my emotional state more than to their desire to connect to and bond with their niece or grandchild . . . *my* baby.

I understand that I am asking for the impossible. That I'm asking them to see needs in me that I can't even see myself. And I can see how I am responsible for creating my own struggle by not communicating it. I'm sure that if I did, they'd thank me for being honest and do whatever they could to help.

This is so difficult for me to write. I'm terrified that the people I love more than anything will not understand that I'm not angry with them. I know they've done absolutely nothing wrong. I adore and appreciate them for creating a world for Pepper where the only experience she has had to date, three months into her life, is having been showered with nonstop love. I don't want anyone to feel that *they* have hurt me. And yet, I have been hurting.

At the same time, I have spoken with many other women who have had this same experience, whether they have children or not, of feeling deeply conflicted and misunderstood. These women don't know how to voice this for their same fears of hurting people they love, and they judge themselves for these feelings they don't even understand.

These complexities, these simultaneously occurring but completely opposite experiences, are the essence of new motherhood and, as I'm realizing, life in general.

If we can't open up the space and experience these emotions in totality, and instead we repress them, then we hold pain, hurt ourselves, and develop misplaced resentment.

And if we can't learn to hold that space for others without taking it personally and being offended by the complexity of someone else's experience, we hold pain, hurt ourselves and develop misplaced resentment.

Just writing this has opened up space for me. As much as it scares me to share, it's essential to fully own our experiences so that we can grow to a deeper level of understanding.

To be understood.

19.
I WANT TO KILL SOMEONE

THE HARDEST MOMENTS are at 7:30 at night when I am changing Pepper, and Opi, my Neapolitan mastiff (picture Fang from *Harry Potter*), is begging for attention to play. I'm tired, Sibe is still at work, and I still need to cook dinner.

And for some reason, this is the time I decide to try to do laundry.

I bash my foot into the changing-table leg trying to retrieve Opi's toy for her.

"FUCK!"

I lose it. In moments like this, I want to scream, break something, and burst into tears.

My anger is masking guilt. Guilt that for the fourth time today, Opi is feeling neglected and desperate for my undivided attention.

Guilt that she's aware that as soon as I throw the toy, I turn back to Pepper on the changing table.

Guilt that as soon as I throw the toy, Pepper is aware of my distraction and stops cooing.

Before that guilt, I was enjoying talking to P and watching her adorable smile light up as she baby-talked back.

I was enjoying Opi's puppy-like pounce as she jumped up onto the bed to catch her toy.

As the game progresses, Opi drops the toy just out of reach. She's begging me to give her my full attention.

I can't. Pepper is naked on the changing table, and I can't walk away.

"Bring it here, Opi."

She doesn't. Instead, she gives me that look that entreats me to come play for real.

I can't. I don't want to. I just want this undivided moment with Pepper. I want to enjoy her adorable smile without knowing and feeling Opi's disappointment.

I want to give Opi the undivided attention that she wants. I want her to not feel displaced, neglected, disappointed.

I want Pepper not to notice when I turn my back to give Opi some half-assed attempt at attention. Who knows, maybe no one but me feels any of this.

I want everyone to go away and not need anything from me, and I want everyone to be closer, more connected and attended to.

It builds. I kick the changing table and it's the last straw.

In that moment, it's just too much.

I hope Pepper can't feel this. I fake a smile and give her a kiss.

Opi sighs and lies down at my feet.

20.

SEND HELP

"I BETTER SEE YOU in the gym twice this week."

Kind and challenging words from a friend who loves me and wants me to own my strength and recover.

"It might be a great idea to start your day with a workout instead of a meditation. I have a mentor who says 'body first.'"

Beautiful advice from a brilliant friend who wants me to focus more on what my body can do than what it can't.

"It gets easier, I promise. I had a friend who had a C-section, and she was back in her routine after four months."

Empathy falling flat.

Three months after my surgery, I can't go to the gym without anger escalating as my workout progresses. In fact, during my last few workouts I found myself listening to ragey heavy metal or trap. This alone should have been a sign that something was wrong. I typically work out to Selena Gomez and Justin Bieber remixes.

Next time you catch me listening to Iron Maiden or Metallica, send help.

It wasn't until a call with a mastermind group several months into motherhood that I was reminded of how angry I still am. And under that, how confused and disoriented I am. Under that, how fucking *sad* I still am.

When I said that I had my entire identity based around not being a mother, what I didn't say was that I saw motherhood as an inferior life path. I was ashamed for people to know I was pregnant. I was terrified that it would ruin my career and derail everything I worked my entire life to create. My entire identity, my entire sense of who I am in this world, was based around the success I was working to create in my business, and channeled into mastering the skill of professional coaching. It wasn't just that I didn't want kids. It was how much I wanted to be *not* a mother.

I didn't even know this myself until I was pregnant. Throughout the seven months of working with my shaman before P's arrival, I was continually astounded at how deeply integrated being "not a mother" was.

I need you to know this so you can have a microscopic understanding of the sense of pain, confusion, anger, and sadness that I keep forgetting is there until it exploded in tears when someone suggested that I start my day with yoga instead of meditation.

The concept of me being a mother was completely out of the realm of possibility for me. So entering the hospital pregnant and leaving with a baby but having missed the delivery . . . is fucking with me. There is something so deeply unfair about missing the moment she was born, the literal transition into motherhood, that I just can't get over.

I was induced. And I was in labor for two and a half days before doctors determined that I needed an emergency C-section when Pepper's heart rate spiked and wouldn't return to normal.

Because my epidural had been injected a millimeter off, only one half of my body was numb. On the operating table, the surgeon was pushing to get things moving, but I could still feel and move half of my lower body.

A split-second decision.

"We have to get this baby out of you fifteen minutes ago. Will you undergo general anesthesia?"

There wasn't a decision to make. I was terrified, confused. "Of course. Put me under. Do whatever you have to."

It wasn't until weeks later that I started to feel the impact of that choice.

I was unconscious for the birth of my daughter. I missed it. So did Sibe, since he wasn't allowed in the operating room.

I didn't meet her for five hours, and when I did, I was so high I barely remember it. I remember waking up the next morning, in a fuzzy daze. I heard the muffled sound of a baby crying. Without moving my head, my eyes shifted left to see a baby in a hospital bed next to me. I felt nothing, numb physically and emotionally.

I would later discover that it was because of the heavy painkillers I was on. But after everything I had been through and all the work I had done to prepare myself emotionally for this moment, it was so painful to see this human that I'd worked so hard to create the capacity to love and then to feel no connection to her.

It wasn't until several months later that I realized how angry I was to have missed the moment of her birth. I was at the gym, and lifting my foot an inch off the floor required so much concentration that it was as frustrating as trying to raise an eyebrow if I'd lost that eyebrow in a surgery I didn't want months before.

The week before my delivery, past my due date, I was in a cycle class and doing squats on the bench I could now not even do a sit-up on. I felt like my strength had been ripped away from me. I was so strong and so fit right up until my delivery. I literally trained my body for labor the way an athlete prepares for game day. I should not have had a C-section.

The moment I would meet Pepper and welcome her into the world was stolen from me. I had visualized that moment more than a hundred times in meditation in preparation for my delivery. No matter what, I'd never get to live that moment. I worked so hard to be ready to become a mother, to transition into a role that I never asked for and didn't want. I worked for months with a shaman and coach to change my mindset around motherhood and heal my ancient pain. I rearranged my business. I spent hours in hypnobirthing classes to prepare to be completely present and conscious during the birth. I went from devastated about being pregnant to excited to be a mother, and I worked harder and more relentlessly than anyone else on the planet to do it.

And the moment of delivery, the moment I would transition from pregnant mother-to-be into mother, was ripped away from me. I lay down on that operating table pregnant and woke up five hours later with a baby I couldn't connect to.

I cannot begin to explain how disorienting and confusing that is for me. When I work out and feel the incapability of my body, I feel all of this in full force: intense anger fueled by disorienting sadness.

I'm convinced my delivery didn't need to get to that point. I'm equally aware that I'll never know for sure and it doesn't serve me to believe that. I'm aware that if I believed the C-section was a true emergency and instead felt thankful that those doctors were there to save our lives, I'd be much happier.

Except I don't.

I've met too many women who have had similar experiences and ended up with C-sections they didn't want. In fact, I was warned by my hypnobirthing instructor that my birth scenario was the exact one likely to occur if I gave birth in a hospital. I rolled my eyes at her internally each time she mentioned it in class and judged her as being too anti-Western medicine.

I don't know what to do with this anger and sadness. Sometimes I completely forget it's there. I wake up cranky and frustrated, and only when I'm in conversation with a friend who innocently suggests working out before meditating does it come pouring out of the depths.

"This might always be a part of you. It will feel less painful over time, but it might always be there," the friend says.

That makes me want to set shit on fire while I blast Metallica out of the speakers of my Jeep.

Then I'm reminded that I'm back in anger because it's so much easier to feel than the sadness it's barely restraining underneath.

The seemingly endless stream of tears restarts. This is how we have to process painful experiences. They have to run their course, and they can't do that when you mask them with heavy metal–fueled, rage-filled productivity. (If I had a twenty for how many times I've learned this . . .) Sure, that may be healthier than setting cars on fire, but it only channels the anger; it doesn't process the pain.

So, that's where I am today. Trying to become more conscious that I (like most people) am avoiding the pain of something I cannot change by masking it with anger and pushing people away with my grumpiness and isolation. I guess I'm grieving.

There's a Buddhist story about a woman who lost her child. She begs the Buddha to help her. He tells her that he can help her, but she has to collect mustard seeds for medicine. She agrees. Before she leaves, he adds that the mustard seeds must come from a house that has not been touched by death. When the woman visits each of the houses to find one that has seeds that might help, she discovers that there is no such house. In seeing that she is not alone in her suffering, she is able to bury her child and release her grief.

In this, I'm reminded that sadness and suffering are not senseless, which is how I feel when I am so angry and sad about this loss. When I am willing to be vulnerable, and have the courage to be witnessed in my pain by friends in those low moments, I receive so much love from them.

Grief and sadness crack us open. When we are brave enough to go into their depths and be momentarily swept away by them over and over until we are no longer subsumed, they allow us to connect more profoundly to others, to ourselves—to expand our capacity for empathy, expand our capacity to receive more love from others, to reach out to and help others.

And in all honesty, that only helps a little right now.

21.
DESIRE AND FRUSTRATION

IT HAS BEEN FASCINATING to watch Pepper learn to crawl. And it's been fascinating to observe myself watching Pepper learn to crawl.

When we go in to wake her up in the morning, she opens her eyes and *immediately* rolls over onto all fours, shifts her hips back, and starts rocking like she's gaining momentum. It happens so fast I wouldn't even be able to reach over to my phone and hit snooze on my alarm in the time she goes from eyes closed to hips rocking.

I noticed this when she was trying to sit up as well. She couldn't help randomly stiffening up her entire body like a plank on her back, over and over. It would almost be compulsive if it weren't natural.

That's exactly what fascinates me about it. It's totally natural. She has this completely innate desire to evolve. Every few weeks, we've watched her repeatedly pushing the limits of her own mobility. She couldn't fight it if she tried.

Despite how frustrated she gets.

This same thing happens in me and just about everyone else

I've ever met. We also have an innate, completely-out-of-our-control desire to evolve. To us, this looks like wanting different things in life. We want better jobs and relationships, more money and travel, etc. This is our version of crawling. We can't not want despite how hard we may try. Watching this unfold so naturally in Pepper helps me see that wanting is what pushes us to evolve.

And in our efforts to grow, to get what we want, we get so frustrated. When Pepper is on all fours, rocking her hips forward and backward like she's winding up to launch, she might build up a couple of reps and then lift both arms and fall flat on her face. She might do it a few times, and I see the frustration build.

I noticed my own desire for her to get it faster. Worrying that if I didn't have her on her tummy enough, she wouldn't learn fast enough. Sometimes I'd try to help her and show her to lift one hand instead of two. But none of it helped. I was only rushing her natural process. She didn't need me to intervene. *I* needed me to intervene because it was tough to watch her little face scrunch in frustration.

I'm fascinated with her frustration. Once I let go of the difficulty of seeing her experience these obstacles, I actually marveled at how natural the dance between desire and frustration are. What if frustration is just *part* of desire? I get frustrated when I'm trying to "crawl" toward something I want. I've always thought that I, and everyone else I know, get frustrated because we're rushing the process, out of integrity with what we say we will do, ungrateful for what we have, stuck on some limiting belief. But what if we're frustrated because frustration is the natural fuel for desire? What if frustration is just the natural force of evolution pushing against where you currently are?

Pepper doesn't have the capacity to be ungrateful yet. She has no concept of being behind. She can't be out of integrity because she doesn't plan to wake up early and work on her crawling and then sleep in. She hasn't even consciously decided that crawling is the next thing she wants. She hasn't had any time to form limiting beliefs about her ability to crawl and what it means about her. So her frustration must be primal.

To see frustration as a natural, primal, and unavoidable part of desire and growth is actually liberating. To see that it's nearly impossible to not want is also liberating. Wanting more doesn't mean you're ungrateful for what you have, and it doesn't mean that what you have isn't enough. It simply means you're wanting—the force of evolution moving through you, preparing you to dance with frustration.

And that wanting will inevitably push you into growing and learning, or, at the very least, taking certain actions that push you a little to get whatever it is you want. And inherent in that process of growing, learning, and acting, you will be frustrated. And it doesn't have to mean anything.

22.

FROM SERIAL KILLER TO SUPERHERO

MONDAY NIGHTS CAN BE HARD. Sibe doesn't get home until eight, and the two hours between five and seven feel like they're three days long sometimes. We've started to call it "mile twenty-five," like the end of a marathon. You're so close to the end but seriously considering tapping out.

Usually, these days I feel like I accomplish about .03 percent of what I set out to do that day. And by the evening, poor Opi is like "Oh, hey, *finally* I can get some attention."

I run through my plan in my head. "P can go down to sleep by seven, and then I can get some writing or work done." As seven approaches, I realize how insanely tired I am and how it's going to be almost impossible to write or do any work that involves more than doing no work at all. Frustration builds. I start to replay and get annoyed at every little thing that distracted me that day.

That I *let* distract me. I'm mad at myself for every wasted moment I was out of my integrity, and I feel my mood drop and start to spiral a little.

I'm irritated that I didn't prepare lunch ahead of time, even though I work from home. I'm mad at Sibe for needing to eat dinner. I'm annoyed that I have to make it. I'm annoyed at Opi for wanting to play because she's been neglected for eight hours. I'm annoyed at her for needing to go outside to poop, so I now have to bundle up a sleepy baby, put her in the stroller, and walk around the fucking block. I'm annoyed that we live in a city and don't have a yard to let her out in. I'm annoyed at Pepper for crying while we're walking because the poor kid is so tired. I'm annoyed that it's winter, and cold, and dark.

I'm mad at myself for scheduling and managing my time so badly, again.

I feel the tension building. About every four days, this feeling rises up inside of me that makes me feel like I could punch a stranger. This feeling, I have come to learn, is a need for a few minutes off and for much more discipline in being *on* when I have help. Sibe and I have come to pay close attention to this feeling in each other. It's met with a swift "What can I get you? Sit down; let me give you a back rub." Which diffuses it almost instantly.

But right now, I'm walking down the cold, dark city streets, waiting for Opi to poop so I can go home. That back rub is hours away.

Finally. Opi is pooping.

Pepper is still crying.

My attempt at a lullaby:

Rock-a-bye Pepper, we're walking a loop.
All over Lawrenceville so Opi will poop
Mommy is losing it inside her head
She cannot wait til everyone is in bed

Some days that's about the best I can do, kiddo.

I'm sure at some point I'll look back on this period of our life and think, "You guys were fucking *killing* it, and also totally insane.

You had a six-month-old baby, you were rebuilding your business, launching a new business together, and working on two books at the same time. What was wrong with you? Also, good job."

There's a Buddhist teaching about the germination of karma. Every seed you plant has a germination period, a length of time required for that seed to mature into a tree.

The part of me that wants to punch strangers would like that germination period to be minutes.

The teaching shares that it's not up to you how quickly the efforts you put in produce results. But you can speed up the germination period by expressing gratitude to *yourself for your efforts* at the end of every day.

This is *so* different from what most people (I) do. So different from my gut reaction to be super annoyed that I only did X. Not only do I not practice gratitude for my efforts, I don't even remember what I have completed. I once rewrote my entire website and then paid my friend twenty dollars for losing our bet that I would not rewrite my website by the time we met again. She kept the money and told me it was a lesson to practice more gratitude for what I accomplished.

I'm so practiced in experiencing a lack of satisfaction in what I accomplish that gratitude for effort is a very foreign concept. So, as I walk home, cold and irritated, baby crying in the stroller, neglected dog faithfully by my side, I give it another attempt.

What did I accomplish today? I created space to bond and snuggle with P in the morning, as I do every morning. I rearranged my career to be present for her and still work close to full time, or at the very least generate enough income to sustain our lifestyle while raising a tiny human. Despite how crazy my world feels right now, I still manage to be present for my clients. Some days I work out, and some days I don't.

I feel my energy shift a little, coming back to the present moment. A few hours earlier, walking Pepper from the car, down the hill to the apartment with the diaper bag on my back, my work bag on my shoulder, and Opi's leash in my hand, I passed the guy who owns the tattoo-removal shop below me. "Hey, Supermom!" he cheerily says, as he has every day since I had Pepper, in a voice with so much authenticity that I believe him for a moment: *I am Supermom.* My heart opens a little more.

A thought enters my mind that makes me laugh: *I guess some days you start feeling like a superhero and some days you end feeling like a serial killer.*

23.
EXPANDING YOUR CAPACITY

LAST NIGHT, LIKE MOST NIGHTS before bed, Pepper was wrapped up in her hooded bath towel, sitting on Sibe's lap on the rocker in her room. Also like most nights, P was mustering all of the strength in her tiny body (which is a *ton*) to bust out of her bath towel and go streaking through the apartment, two fingers in her mouth and giggling and shrieking the whole time, marveling in delight at her own escape.

Sibe used all of *his* strength, and a French frog named Pierre, to keep her on his lap. Pierre is our bedtime hero. He's dating Fancy the flamingo, and most nights, the interactions of the French frog, accent done by me, and the southern flamingo, part played by Sibe, entertain Pepper long enough to outlast her desire to flee and wind herself up so much that she can't fall asleep.

The last, chaotic thirty minutes of Pepper's day, on the wrong day, can be enough to make me and Sibe want to flee the scene and go streaking through the house, but more in the "I've completely lost my mind" way than the "nine-month-old baby giggling and shrieking" kind of way.

But most nights, it's magical. The chaos and fatigue are dwarfed by the absolute joy that it is to soak in Pepper, alternating between giggling hysterically and popping her two fingers into her mouth and plopping her head down onto Sibe's chest as she starts to get tired, and then popping back up three seconds later and peeking over the side of the chair again to see if Pierre is still slowly sneaking across the floor to snuggle-attack her.

A scene that is often interrupted by Opi trying to snag Pierre just before he reaches Pepper by biting one of Pierre's long, mint-green legs as they flail by her. When I tell her no, she usually retreats to find her shell of a blue hippo that she previously ripped all of the stuffing and squeaker out of for me to throw down the hallway to fetch. It's in the moments of the most joy and laughter with P that Opi most wants to play.

Months ago, that request was enough to drive me to rage. The moments where Pepper is giggling and Opi wants to play historically have been maddening for me. Like so many other women I've talked to about this, initially you feel a twinge of frustration—"Not now, Opi"—followed by a subtle pang of guilt for realizing that this is the hundredth day in a row where you've said "Not now, Opi." The relentlessness of the requests then start to weigh on you, and the frustration and guilt start to amass energy and momentum, and within seconds to minutes you feel a full-on-tantrum-level rage that makes you want to just scream and freak out.

I *want* to be completely present with Pepper *and* give Opi attention. I *want* to give my entire self to my work *and* never miss a second with Pepper. I *want* to be intimately connected to Sibe *and* immersed in the chaos of parenthood with two career-driven people. All of those things are equal parts of me. And the times where they're all requesting me in the same moment, I feel like I'm being drawn and quartered.

But last night, something was different. I didn't get to that point. Just as Opi entered the scene and shoved her blue hippo into my lap as she always does, the moment that would normally trigger the initial frustration and put me on the path to internal rage, something else happened.

I zoomed out.

Normally, I'm trying desperately to savor the moment with Pepper. To soak in that adorable baby giggle, to permanently capture the image of her as a baby, sitting in Sibe's lap in her bath towel. I know one day (feels like tomorrow) she's going to be an adult, and we'll be trying to remember these moments, so I try desperately to be as present as possible to savor each one completely.

Simultaneously, I've been on a hunt to understand that experience of frustration, guilt, and rage since it first happened to me just days into Pepper's life.

That night, when I zoomed out, I understood it much more profoundly. In my *desperate* attempt to savor the moment with Pepper and to be *completely* present with her, I was blocking my ability to be *totally* present with the moment as a whole. My desire to be completely present was actually what was dividing me. Feeling divided causes the initial frustration. That feeling of "I can't attend to Pepper without ignoring Opi" (substitute *present for Pepper and ignoring work*, or *present with work and ignoring Pepper*, or *present with Opi and ignoring Sibe*, etc. ad infinitum). Being constantly pulled in opposite directions at once and the impossibility of meeting all of those simultaneous requests and my *desire* to do so quickly escalates into the rage.

But I saw in that moment that it wasn't the parts of my life that were causing me to feel divided. I was just too zoomed in on one *aspect* of that moment. I was zoomed in on Pepper's face, the sound of her giggling, the feeling of savoring it all.

But when I zoomed out to take in the *total* moment, I noticed the early summer–sunset light pouring through the window, I saw a young family, a loving but tired dad, a mother in love with her husband and baby, *and* I saw a loving and giant dog who wanted to be a part of that moment, throwing her massive paws around as if knocking to get in, to add to the playfulness by playing herself.

When I zoomed out, I didn't see a woman who was playing with her dog and as a result missing the moment with her giggling baby. I saw a woman immersed in the totality of a beautiful moment full of moving but integrated parts.

I zoomed out; I expanded. My capacity grew.

Initially, I understood the word *capacity* as "the ability to hold," and I was always trying to expand my capacity to hold more. But in exploring the deeper, even earlier root of the word, I learned it also means "to grasp." Instead of trying to grasp parts of these moments, or grasp parts of my life, or desperately trying to grasp on to the moments because I know they're fleeting—grasping like a verb, an action you take with your hands—I'm grasping now in the sense of an understanding. Capacity is not about expanding to hold more, do more, and do better. Expansion of your capacity is not about taking *on* more *in* your life; it's about taking *in* more *of* your life.

24.
LOOK UP

LOOK UP, I THOUGHT. In the moment, it felt much like any other thought.

That's the trick, the trap, and the key.

I looked up. First, I noticed that the trees, lit up by the sunrise, looked like they were on fire with golden light.

Then, just in time, I noticed a spiderweb with several dead bugs at eye level, a millisecond away from being in my eyes.

Like Morpheus from *The Matrix* at a backyard lawn party, I instantly limboed my way under just in time to avoid an embarrassing overreactive dance involving spastically petting myself and screaming to get two already dead bugs off of me.

But that wasn't the point.

Look up, the thought had urged. And I did.

In the exact moment I needed to. To catch something beautiful and miss something awful.

I literally stopped on the trail in awe and bewilderment. I looked up at the sky, as if I expected to see a handful of pleased and amused, and probably surprised, faces hanging down over the edges of the morning clouds, chattering amongst themselves: "Well, would you look at that? She's finally listening."

"I told you the gold trees would get her. Didn't I tell you? I told you the gold would light up that web just in time!"

"Did you SEE that *Matrix* move she pulled? Next time let's let her hit the web. I bet that would be hilarious."

But that voice didn't come from floating heads in the clouds.

When I walked into the park where Opi and I have been coming every morning, I felt stuck in my head—already normalized to the beauty of this place and the music of the forest at sunrise, the dozens of different birds singing against the background of a running stream and the percussion of a well-timed woodpecker in the distance—and afraid because my husband insisted I carry a knife, leaving me waiting for some invisible threat.

I was headed to the same spot I always go to sit and write when a thought, not that different from any other thought at first glance, said, *Hike. What's the difference between my inner voice and a random thought?* I thought in an instant attempt to rationalize myself away from this request (command?).

If you have to ask that, you know the answer, I thought.
Damn it. I'll hike.
But quickly. I need to write. That's why I'm here, I thought.

This place inside, the one that told me to look up, is the same place that told me to hike. It's also the same place that for two *years* has been saying, *Spend your mornings in nature*. It's the same place that committed me to seven sunrise hikes in seven days.

And it's the place that the words I'm writing now are coming from.

But you don't get access unless you listen.

And the requests that this place makes are often confusing, incomplete, and absolutely inconvenient.

But they're never wrong.

You show up to the park to write, but that voice tells you to hike first. And then you discover the perfect inspiration to write.

You're in the middle of a workday, stressed and busy, and it tells you to go for a walk. And you solve the challenge you've been struggling with for weeks.

You're in an argument with your husband, and it tells you to apologize, and you diffuse the tension.

You're walking out of your sister's house, and it tells you to go give a hug, a real hug, to your brother-in-law. And you two hug for real for the first time.

We hear so much about this voice in life-saving moments. "I was about to board the plane and something told me not to and the plane crashed!" In reality, this voice is much more subtle than that.

Sometimes you hear it just in time to save you, from a plane crash or a spiderweb on a hike.

But most of the time, it's whispering suggestions not to save your life but to create your life.

It's the same voice that, without saying anything, let me know I was having this baby. No other option.

The one that, early on in P's life, as I lay next to Sibe, longing for Pepper, showed me the default future ahead of me if I didn't expand.

The one that knew this book had to be written. The one that gives me strange commands like *Now run. Hike the trail again.* And then steps in with the perfect words to pour onto paper.

It's the voice you're ignoring right now that's asking you to listen— giving you confusing, incomplete, and absolutely inconvenient ideas.

Move to Hawaii.

Leave your boyfriend.

Start that makeup business.

Travel.

Marry him. Now leave him.

You might hear these calls. But you might not be able to hear them yet. You also have to listen to the more subtle ones, the ones that almost feel like it wouldn't make a difference if you listened or not. It does. These are the ones that matter the most. They're the ones that teach you to listen. To trust them.

When you listen, these are the ideas that create your life.

Not the one you have.

The one you want.

25.

WILD

I'M COMING A-L-I-V-E.

Like *really* alive. It feels like there's someone else inside of me tearing her way out to the surface. Sometimes it scares me and I want to push her back down.

But more often, I want to un*leash* her. She's *wild*. Scary, almost. But scary in a way that is sexy. Untamed.

She's me.

She scares Sibe. He's afraid she'll leave him. She reads books called *Untamed*. And he looks at me, nervous. But he's *so* wrong. She wants him, all of him, more of him. Endlessly. He brings her even more to life. She wants to grab his hand and sprint into their life, twirling, falling to the ground laughing.

She wants to dance. All the time. But when she dances, she doesn't follow a video. She doesn't use choreography like I did in college. She *feels* the music and it releases her. The more she feels it, the more she moves. And when she gets a taste of freedom, it sets her on fire, and the flames burn wild. She is the flames, the heat, the fire. And she's *wild*. Devastatingly wild.

She's impatient. But in the way of someone imprisoned for a lifetime who knows freedom is imminent. The energy of freedom fills their soul, p-u-s-h-i-n-g them out of the prison doors.

And she's expansive. Massive. Endless. Limitless. Free.

And she's happy. She can't stop smiling. She's so happy to be free. She adores life. The lines between her and life are blurred. You can't tell where she starts and life begins.

For thirty years, I didn't trust her. She got me into trouble. In sixth grade, my art teacher asked me to write a letter to her about what I loved about art class. This wild me told the truth. She wrote a letter explaining why she shouldn't have to write the letter. That art class was miserable and the teacher was mean. We got sent to the principal's office and I had to apologize.

In second grade, she ran away from day camp and talked her friends into coming with her, and they got lost in the trees near the school for hours. Even then, she knew they were fine. She stared in defiance at the school counselor towering over her, scolding her for chasing her freedom.

In high school and college, she dove headfirst into her feelings for the men who used her body and discarded her heart. And she followed her heart into the pain over and over. Always trusting. Hair on fire, she charged into life, into her desires, and into love. She never thought twice about being herself. And she was hit from all sides with discipline, heartbreak, and rejection. She just kept throwing her wild into the unknown. She didn't care.

But I did. It hurt; I hurt. And I buried her to keep myself safe. But safety has made me numb. And now I'm letting her out.

I'm not just letting her out. I'm unleashing her wildness into the world. Into my world. And allowing her to take it over. To take me over. To let everything that's not me fall away forever. The weight, the clothes, the city I live in. None of it is her. And my life, my spirit, and my body are hers to claim.

She has a ferociousness that would scare me if it didn't excite me so much. She wants to tear out of her prison like a wild animal. The feeling is indescribable. Elation. A kind of joy I've never felt. I almost feel insane. I want to laugh so hard that I cry—where I can't tell if I'm laughing or crying.

The more I feel her, the more I want to reach inside of myself, grab her by the forearm, and pull her out of the depths and thrust her out ahead of me, twirling, dancing, and laughing to lead my life, raise my daughter, coach my clients, and love my husband.

Take it, all of it, I say to her. *Make it yours.*

26.

MAMA NEEDS A NEW SPORTS BRA

I'M ALWAYS SO SURPRISED by how much there is to see when you really look at something. Recently with a client, I had her stare at my yellow coffee mug with a giraffe on it for several minutes to tell me what she saw. Initially she was confused by the assignment, but she went along anyway. She was then astounded by how much there was to notice beyond "yellow mug with a giraffe." She noticed the subtle shades of yellow created by the black outlining the giraffe's features, the detail in the facial expression, that it was actually a pretty great drawing of a giraffe, the hairs on the chin, and the things on its head. We laughed as she paused her analysis and said, "I should really look up what those are called."

The longer we look at something, the more nuance we see. This is as true when studying some aspect of ourselves as it is when analyzing a yellow coffee mug with a giraffe on it. You can see detail and inconsistencies that you may not have noticed, and most importantly, this often leads to curiosity and action. *"I should really look up what those are called."*

When acted upon, curiosity almost always leads to expansion. I have been in the practice of looking at myself, like my client looked at that goofy giraffe, since the day I discovered I was pregnant. But it never ceases to amaze me how much I have completely been missing until I sit down and stare at it.

Last night, I sat on my couch with my new visual-branding coach, both of us staring at the evidence of my personal style—more specifically, my style expression, or lack thereof. Somehow over the last four years, I've migrated to wearing all-black athletic clothes every day. I can't even blame motherhood; I had given up the habit of taking care of myself long before Pepper came around. I'm not even 100 percent sure I was ever really in the habit.

But a few things occurred recently that hinted that it was time to sit down and stare. First, I bought a forty-dollar handmade romper for Pepper to wear on her first birthday. Considering that she will probably wear this thing twice, I think that's a lot of money. I also have not yet purchased anything for *me* to wear on her first birthday. It feels like too much, unnecessary. *But wait, am I not also turning one? Shouldn't I dress to celebrate myself as well?* But I couldn't bring myself to do it.

The other thing that occurred was my shaman made a completely harmless remark that led to an embarrassing revelation, then a powerful revelation, then an internal revolution. He said, "Your content is high vibe, but you're in your 'mom clothes.' It doesn't match." He was referring to my social media presence and lack of personal brand. It was bad enough to be called out for looking like a bum presenting my professional content, but it was even worse because these *weren't* my "mom clothes." They were just my clothes.

So, I sat down and started staring. What I saw first was something unbelievable. For so long, I thought I would consider myself as having "made it" when I looked online and saw myself as equal with so many of the coaches I admire. I invest tens of thousands of dollars a year and countless hours to grow my skills professionally to be able to "compete" at this level. I always felt frustrated that I just couldn't figure out what the gap was. Why did I feel I always had to work harder to compete when I could perform at a similar, or higher, level? Why didn't people see me at the same level? I felt like a Honda Civic with a Ferrari engine, frustrated that no one could see my power or beauty when they looked at me.

It never occurred to me until that moment, though, that I was competing so hard on talent, using it to overcompensate for image, when I could just also work on my image. As I stared longer, I saw that style, clothes, hair, and makeup were something I always considered frivolous and for an elusive "later." In fact, I kind of scoffed internally any time I read something about "taking care of yourself as a woman." I judged it as juvenile and then self-righteously commended myself for taking care of myself in ways that "really counted," like integrity, investing in coaching, and having solid boundaries, somehow finding it of higher spiritual value not to wash my hair.

As I stared at this even longer with curiosity, I discovered that this was something I picked up in high school. Going to a wealthy, mostly white high school full of girls who looked like Regina George, I never felt I could compete. In high school, being "hot" was the ultimate prize. I just couldn't look like a blonde, skinny, rich girl. So, internally, I started to compete in the only ways I felt I could. I could be smarter, a better human, and more successful. Eventually they would see that I won.

Except, seventeen years later, I'm the only one still competing. And I haven't won yet. And being smart, a good person, and a successful coach still hasn't made up for feeling like I'm not a skinny, blonde, rich girl.

So, there I sat on my couch, staring at my lack of personal style expression and a forty-dollar romper for my almost one-year-old, and I shared with my friend and newly hired style coach that I don't even own a sports bra younger than five years. My sports bras are five times older than my kid, and the only real bra I own is a nursing bra, which I was immediately informed did not count. For some reason, of all the shit I've shared in this book, this is hands down one of the most embarrassing.

But this is also the way expansion works as a human being. We kind of exist in emotional layers. We have our very deep, personal (and universal) experiences, those that exist kind of in the middle, and our external, which I judged as shallow but are actually only surface-level layers.

I have spent the last nineteen months doing expansive work on the deepest experiences of my spiritual and emotional being. I've explored the "middle" ground, and now, those things feel solid. The ground no longer feels like it's crumbling under my feet. I feel happy 98 percent of the time, and even when I'm down, I don't stay there. Sibe and I can dance through intensely challenging relationship evolutions and even pandemics. Financial fluctuations and painful global events don't bring me down for long.

"How would you describe your current style?" my new style coach asked me.

"Backpacker who shops in a lost-and-found bin," I replied. We both laughed.

The tectonic plates of my being have shifted and are bringing to the ground everything on the surface that isn't sound.

One by one we went through the items in my closet. My coach lovingly teased me, inquired with concern as to why I still have a shirt that doesn't fit and has a hole in it, and encouraged Pepper to "wave bye-bye" to it as I tossed it into a pile representing a part of me that no longer exists.

27.

BEAUTIFUL AND LETHAL

NINE MONTHS INTO PEPPER'S LIFE, Sibe and I were going to bed. He said, "This is life now, isn't it? It's not going to slow down, is it?" I told him my guess is that it might only speed up. He replied, "We have to connect more. I don't want us to get lost in the busyness."

My mind jumped immediately to a moment right after P was born that was the impetus to write this book, when I saw that default future. He was right, but this time I didn't have the fear and guilt that I felt in the moments after she was born. There is such unity, love, and support in the way we parent Pepper. Sibe and I have always made the best team. "Can I do anything for you?" is a question we ask each other five times a day.

We also love to do everything together. In the morning, we literally race each other into Pepper's room giggling to wake her up together. She wakes to the sound of laughter every single morning. He gives her a bath at night in the kitchen sink while I cook dinner. He cleans up while I give her her bottle, and then we sit together before bed at night while he makes her laugh before putting her down to sleep. And then we collapse on the couch, exhausted, for two hours before bed.

There is so much love in our teamwork that I almost missed something both beautiful and lethal.

Lying in bed with Sibe that night, it occurred to me that we were back in that initial fearful moment, together. Pepper was in her own bed in the other room, but all of *our* energy was directed toward her.

Becoming a parent is one of the wildest experiences. There's a selfishness that I crave from pre-parenting. Every day revolved around me. *What do I want? How am I suffering? What do I need?* I laugh as I consider a craving for my "old" suffering. Once you become a parent, there is this tiny, adorable little black hole in your life that pulls in everything that gets close.

Pepper's massive gravitational force was pulling all of the love, attention, and energy that Sibe and I possessed toward her. The trap is that it feels both necessary and good for it to go there. Until you're lying in bed aware of how little is left for each other.

Another moment to remind me what this journey is about. Expansion.

It would be easy to feel despair and fear in that moment, like I did that night I decided to use this journey for expansion. But I don't feel that fear and dread now. I've been practicing expansion for nine months, and I've learned that when fear is most present and you feel most constricted, those are the moments to expand. And it's a choice—the unmarked, barely visible path easily overshadowed by the more obvious path of fear.

At that moment early on, I made a choice. But until Sibe's confession, it hadn't occurred to me that we'd also have to learn to expand as a couple. That we'd have to learn not to direct *less* energy to Pepper, but rather to expand our capacity to love each other more *as* we direct energy toward Pepper.

I shared all of this with Sibe. He is used to my reflective and somewhat manic stream of thoughts right before bed, and he sleepily but appreciatively responded.

Life has its own momentum. Default futures are created by unconsciously getting caught up in the current of the life you created. You forget that your desires and actions were the creators of the thing you're experiencing. Once you create something, you become less of the puppet master and more of the puppet to the very play you created. You fall into unconsciousness and make the same choices on autopilot day after day. One day, you wake up in a default future and aren't quite sure how you arrived there.

When Sibe and I moved to Pittsburgh seven years ago, it was never our intention to stay. It was meant to be a short pause as we regrouped from three years of living nomadically all over the world. We made the conscious choice that we wouldn't leave until we felt grounded, opposite of our previous habit of moving to a new city or country every time we felt restless, which led to living in about fifteen countries in three years.

Now in Pittsburgh, we were dangerously close to waking up twenty years later wondering why we never left. This is the pull of the default future. It's created by ignoring the moments like we were having in bed that night—subtle feelings of disconnection excused by being tired, dismissed by promising yourself that you'll address it the next day. You never feel like you're sacrificing anything major until the accumulation of those tiny sacrifices plants you in the exact life you swore you'd never live.

I was nine months into creating an intentional life as a mother and wife, and it had opened my heart and mind in ways I never anticipated. That night woke me to the reality that it was time to channel that same intention back into our relationship to create our combined future.

And the only way to create an intentional future is to access choice in the present moment. This is why when we postpone paying attention to the subtle cues of disconnection until "tomorrow," that feeling of future resolution creates complacency in the present moment, allowing us to ignore the issue. Repeating this day after day doesn't actually create a default future so much as it creates a repeat present that somewhere in the future you have finally had enough of. Only it feels a thousand times worse because you've lived the same disappointing moment compounded over years—knowing all along, on a deeper level, that it wasn't enough.

I refuse to live into that reality with Sibe.

"Relationship bliss does not sit on a mountain top waiting for you to climb up to it. It sits on your shoulder waiting for you to notice it"—a quote from *The Couple's Tao Te Ching*.

In the moments where we notice this disconnection, it's so easy to get sucked into the logistics of our life. How do we organize our life to manage our energy so that there is some energy left to be connected to one another? I could hire a nanny, hire a new coach to increase my income to pay for that nanny, and move into a bigger house so that nanny has space to watch Pepper, all as a path to making space to have more energy to connect to my husband so we don't end up in a default future, or repeat present, of a marriage with no intimacy or connection.

Or we could connect. In the exhaustion of the present moment. Slow down in the chaos long enough to marvel at the energy flying in a thousand different directions, all vying for our complete attention. We can give our complete attention to each other inside all of it at any moment we choose.

I choose this one.

28.

DIVIDE AND BE CONQUERED

I WAS AT DINNER WITH A FRIEND, sharing my thoughts on how if you try to conquer parenthood by dividing yourself, you'll die.

Logistically, you can handle it. It's a lot, but you can do it.

It's the energy and presence required to be a parent that I find the most demanding and the most draining.

But it's impossible when you try to divide.

Dividing looks like holding Pepper and laughing as Opi comes up to shove a toy into my lap. I get frustrated because both of them need something at once.

Dividing looks like trying to check emails while Pepper figures out how the block fits into the hole. And then tries to grab my phone out of my hand a million times and then finally succeeds in knocking over my coffee cup.

Divide and conquer follows that strategy.

It leads to nothing good when you're doing it to yourself. At the end of the day you feel like shit because you've been everywhere and nowhere all at the same time. You've done everything and nothing all day long. It feels like you've let everyone down, most of all yourself. Achieved nothing and enjoyed even less.

"You absolutely cannot divide yourself in parenthood," I shared. "What I've come to find is that the only real way to do it all, and to enjoy it, is to expand. It's just not possible to divide yourself the way you'd need to."

She asked how one expands. "Practically, what do you actually do?"

I paused. I hadn't thought about it so directly until this moment.

"It's more about insight than action," I began. I paused again, longer this time. "It's like you're out to dinner with friends and you're having incredible conversation and then the waitress comes to the table. It breaks the energy for a moment. That's kind of like parenting. There is always something showing up to break the energy. So she leaves and you get back to the conversation. Maybe it takes a moment or two to resync, but you do. You don't let it ruin the meal that the server, a part of dining out, interrupted your flow. The same is true in parenting. Life interrupts and creates chaos because that's what life does. If you don't get too bent out of shape about it, you find your flow a moment or two later.

"Then the food comes. And the food is so good that you completely forget about the conversation. But the incredible food doesn't make the conversation any less great. It's just that your attention is all on the food. That's like loving Opi and Pepper, or Opi and my job, or Pepper and Sibe. But after a few bites, you look up and see your friends enjoying their food. And you notice how perfect the temperature is, and a gorgeous soft breeze blows your hair slightly. And the conversation resumes while you're enjoying each bite. All of a sudden, the entire moment swallows you. You notice the music, the chatter of the tables around you, and the perfect ambience of the restaurant. That's expansion." I paused again, thoughtfully, and sipped my sparkling rosé. "I guess the only difference is that your food doesn't need anything from you."

We both laughed.

"That must be hard, though," she offered, both compassionate and contemplative.

"It is hard." I searched for the right words. "But it's much harder when you don't."

I realize that my expansion had previously been focused on my capacity to hold more. More love for Sibe, Pepper, and Opi. More forgiveness and acceptance and acknowledgment of my own parents, and more ability to get more done, be a better coach, and expand our vision for our life. It was about doing more, being more, and holding more.

But this explanation of the restaurant made me see something magical. Expansion isn't about expanding my capacity to hold more love and life in me. It's really about the ability to be swallowed by life, the life happening around me.

Not to observe the moments of my life, but to experience them as a part of them. Not to try to get more done and master motherhood and professional life, but to experience the dance between them. It's not about holding the moments. It's about letting the moments hold me.

29.

NO SUCH THING AS "DAD GUILT"

GIVEN HOW MUCH MOTHERHOOD was not on my radar, I'm actually surprised at how many ideas about motherhood I'd picked up, let alone taken on as truth. It's not until I fall victim to these ideas that I even know they're there.

I remember standing in our room in our loft-style apartment just a few weeks after Pepper was born and looking at Sibe playing with Pepper's feet as she lay on her back on the couch. A thought popped into my head: *There's no such thing as "dad guilt."* It surprised me. I had already experienced mom guilt a few times. A few other memories came to mind at the same moment, of friends sharing experiences where they felt guilty spending a day at a training, or staying at lunch a little longer because they felt they couldn't leave their husband with the kids an extra hour because he'd get stressed. Occasionally I'll have a conversation with a mother who escaped the trap of feeling guilty for leaving but then feels guilty that she doesn't feel guilty.

There's a strange badge-of-honor look you get from other

mothers that's kind of a "welcome to the club" eyebrow raise, with a hint of a shoulder shrug of resignation.

But every time I experienced it early on, it didn't sit right with me.

Guilt is a waste of energy. And mom guilt isn't a real thing. Don't get me wrong, it's definitely a thing that thousands of women experience. I just don't think it's a thing that happens *to* you because you now have a child.

I think I experienced it because I heard over and over that I would (should?). I witnessed so many other people experiencing it that I assumed it was inevitable. In other words, I experienced it because I expected it.

When I tried to explain the concept to Sibe, he absolutely couldn't get it. Partially because he's a man, partially because he's Dutch, and partially because when you really think about it, it doesn't make sense.

Why exactly should I feel guilty for wanting space to myself? Why should I feel guilty for not wanting every second of every day to be about another human being? Why should I feel guilty for still having the same passions and identity as I had before I "became" a mother? Why should I feel guilty for asking for help, or not being present enough sometimes, or getting frustrated when Pepper wakes up in the middle of the night, or being emotionally unavailable to just about anyone who needs me when I'm too tired?

I just don't buy it. And I refuse to buy *into* it.

I have a theory that guilt, like anxiety, isn't necessarily an emotion in itself. It's a hodgepodge of other emotions that are all experienced at once and get confused, mixed up, and expressed as guilt or anxiety.

When I feel anxious, it's usually a mix of feeling frustrated with myself for not doing something I wanted to do, fearful that I won't achieve something I want to because of it, and angry for not being "there" already. So many different things can look like guilt. "I feel guilty for leaving Pepper" can really mean "I'll miss her." "I feel guilty for needing a break" can mean "I'm tired and I wish I had more capacity right now." "I feel guilty that I can't be more present for you" means "There are two people (experiences) that I want to be present for, and can't."

When it comes to my own "mom guilt," I have found two things. First, sometimes I feel it just because I thought it was a thing that would just happen to me that I couldn't change. When I see this, it's usually enough to let it go and be honest in admitting that I actually don't feel guilty.

Second, this guilt shows up when I want two things that feel like they're in opposition. I want to be fully present for Pepper *and* I want to work. I want to be with Pepper, and I want to go on vacation without her. I want to be a loving, caring parent, and I want to fucking sleep a full night. I want to spend every possible second with Pepper so I don't miss one moment, and I want to work out when I feel like it, even if she's awake.

This conflict creates tension, and I internalize that tension as guilt.

When I can see that, I can do four things. First, I can confront the fact that the two things I want can't happen at the same time, i.e. going on vacation without Pepper can't happen at the same time as going on vacation *with* Pepper. I can accept that I will miss her. A friend once said to me, "How beautiful to miss her." And she said it with such awe and magic that it instantly shifted my experience.

Second, I can expand my experience to see how the conflict is actually a gift. I want to spend every second with Pepper, and I want to work. I'd ask myself how working instead of hanging out with Pepper actually creates more connection between us. I am not just Pepper's mother today. I am Pepper's mother for the rest of her life. And although in this moment her preference might be that I am by her side 100 percent of the time (and I can't even know that with complete certainty), someday she will prefer a mother who has her own life, fulfillment, and who she looks to for inspiration. I can't just become that mother in some instant in the future. I have to cultivate myself as a whole, happy, and fulfilled human *now*. Not to mention, I'm simply happier when I get to do work I love. And when I'm happier, I'm more connected to Pepper.

Third, I can look for a way to blend the things in conflict. I want to work out and also hang out with Pepper. I bought a jogging stroller. I hadn't been into running for a while, but it was an easy way to merge exercise and P time.

Lastly, I can analyze how I am making one thing mean something else that isn't true. I want to sleep a full night and be a loving, caring parent. Being frustrated that she woke up again has nothing to do with me not being loving or caring. It makes me human. I can be frustrated that she's awake and still wake up to feed her. That makes me caring. I care about sleep and I care about Pepper.

The longer you look at something, the more you see. I spent most of my life feeling my emotions and reacting to them. As I've grown deeper (vs. older), I see that the longer I look at my emotional experience, the more nuanced it gets. Emotions result from a mix of thoughts arising from an experience. It's like driving down the highway looking out your window. First, all you see is green. If you slow down, you see a forest. Slow down even more and you see individual trees. If you stop your car, get out, and walk, you can see the individual branches and leaves. Walk up under the tree, lie down, and stare, and you can see different shades of green, the veins in the leaves, the way the brown branch slowly transitions to the small green stem that connects the leaf to the branch.

When we do this with our emotional experience, the more granular we get, the more choice we have. The choice available in how you experience anything is a function of how *slowly* you're moving.

All of this has resulted in a rule I now follow religiously. The worse I feel, and the faster I feel I need to go, the more I slow down.

30.
MOTHERHOOD IS(N'T) HARD

SIBE AND I WERE DRIVING to Virginia for a five-day trip with friends. Pepper stayed with my parents. We were driving just outside of DC, about three and a half hours from our house, and I was looking out the window, which I had down—which drives Sibe crazy on the highway because of how loud it is, but I love the warm summer air on my face, blowing my hair all over the place. It was a beautiful May afternoon, and the trees just outside of DC always seem extra green and lush to me. I felt relaxed. *Really* relaxed. It had been four months since we had an overnight break from parenting, and it felt really good.

"I feel like a human again," I said to Sibe. The words had barely left my mouth and already felt off. He didn't catch it, but I felt it, subtly.

I've said it before. And I've heard it a million times from other parents. But what does that mean? "I feel like a human again." I sat with it longer. I felt relaxed. It felt nice to be off work. But mostly it just felt nice to not direct a constant stream of energy and attention on the wellbeing of another human being. That felt true.

On the surface, "I feel like a human again" is a harmless enough thing to say. But when you put it into the category of all the other "harmless" things we say about motherhood and the frequency with which we repeat them, they feel less harmless to me.

When I was pregnant, I was talking to a friend of mine who had a two-year-old. She said, "Motherhood is just hard." I can't remember the context of why she said it, but it stood out because it wasn't the first time she had said it to me.

Shortly after I had Pepper, I connected with another friend who was exhausted and said, "Motherhood is so dehumanizing."

These phrases aren't harmless. What we often think of as a description of an experience is actually more like an incantation. A phrase that we repeat so often that we're no longer only describing the experience we just *had*, we're *creating* the experiences we're going to continue having.

I was at a dinner party about four months after Pepper was born, sitting at a table of women, half tuned in to the conversation, half letting my mind wander, when one of the women snapped my attention back to the conversation by saying, "My kids are assholes." I was appalled. I wish I could say that my response was more enlightened, but the truth is, she looked disgusting to me at that moment. I actually had a hard time looking at her face while she was talking.

It bothered me so much because her kids aren't assholes. I don't even know them, but I know they're young. It bothered me because I don't even believe *she* thinks her kids are assholes. It bothered me because I think it's a thing she felt she was supposed to say. You're supposed to talk badly about your kids with other women. To complain, to live this role of the martyred mother. And it disgusts me. It wasn't really *her* that disgusted me; it was her fulfilling this cultural habit that did. I would never describe Pepper that way to someone, for the same reason I would never describe my husband as useless, the way many women complain and joke about their husbands.

Because Pepper isn't an asshole; Sibe isn't useless. And more importantly, I don't want to experience them that way even if I sometimes don't like their behavior. Sometimes we see what is there, and sometimes we see what we're told we should see. And sometimes we see what we repeat out loud over and over and prime ourselves to expect.

We think we describe what we see, but the truth is, we see what we describe.

If I repeat that "I feel like a human" when I'm away from Pepper, subconsciously I'll start to feel *dehumanized* when I'm with her. It's more accurate to say what is true—that I'm tired because committing a constant stream of energy to the wellbeing of another human is tiring.

Motherhood isn't dehumanizing.

Kids aren't assholes, and husbands aren't useless.

And motherhood isn't hard.

It's not *not* hard, but when we repeat these phrases to describe ourselves, other people, and experiences, we turn them into permanent objects that we react to the same way over and over instead of fluid experiences that are ever changing. Getting caught up in four months of parenting without a break makes you forget how relaxing it can feel to have someone else care for your kid, but I also recall not feeling completely relaxed all the time before Pepper was born. I stressed out as much then as I do now. Just for different reasons.

It's so important to watch your mouth. To carefully use your language to describe what's true, *and* what you want to experience. The words you use to describe your experience create how you *feel* about it. How you feel about it influences the actions you take that later play a role in what experiences follow. You can begin to see how this can loop back on itself, either positively or negatively.

Motherhood is full of unique, complex, and incredible challenges. It's tough to figure out how to balance your time and energy. Childcare is expensive; it adds a new dimension to your marriage. Being in a group of people with your baby completely divides your presence, making it tough to socialize, and you experience utterly new emotional aspects of yourself.

Yes, motherhood presents all of these challenges, but motherhood as a thing isn't hard. I can only speak for me, but "hard" is not a label I am willing to use to create my experience of motherhood.

As many challenges as it presents, it presents equal moments of absolute bliss. And when we say things like "Motherhood is hard" on repeat, we see all of these moments *through* this lens. At any moment, I could see Pepper pooping in her bed the morning we're leaving for our trip as hard, or hilarious. I might run her to the tub to get the poop off her feet, only to find that in my rush to get her *out* of the bath the night before, I forgot to clean the poop out of the tub. So now I'm holding my squirming, poop-covered ten-month-old in one hand while I try to clean the poop out of the tub with my left hand. Hard, or hilarious? I could see my exhaustion as dehumanizing, or I can realize I'm tired and in need of a break. I could see my kids as assholes or as tiny humans responding to a world that makes absolutely no sense to them. I could see my husband as a man-child, my errand boy, or my best friend.

How I see all of these things dictates how I will respond and react to all of these things. How I see them depends on how I *habitually* describe them.

My quest to fully evolve into motherhood and be able to say "I am a mother" without a tiny internal cringe depends on the way I see and experience motherhood without all of the preconceived ideas about it and the way I make it my own. Until I learn to describe it differently, I won't experience it differently.

31.
I KNOW NOTHING

IN MY HEAD, my plan to finish my book this week was well laid out.

In reality, Pepper turned into a toddler overnight and ruined the entire thing. Aside from rejecting her entire sleep schedule, her time awake consists of throwing 200 tantrums an hour, resisting every single thing you try to do with her, and walking around like an adorable chubby destructo-bot, chucking shit off the table, ripping books from the shelf, and picking fights with Opi.

Within the span of twenty minutes, she pulled hair out of Opi's back leg, pooped on the carpet, and peed on my lap.

I guess it's only appropriate that she throws me a massive motherhood challenge right as I intended to peacefully close out this journey. But seriously, where the fuck did my adorable little angel baby go? Erase everything you've read up until this point. I know nothing.

Also, please send help.

32.
NOT JUST ME AND P ANYMORE

I RECENTLY BECAME AWARE of a fascinating phenomenon called microchimerism. I have no idea how to say this word. It's like when I read Harry Potter and pronounced Hermione as "haar-mee-own" until I saw the movie. I pronounce *microchimerism* as "micro-chromerism," in case you want an incorrect way to say it to yourself.

So, micro-chromerism is the phenomenon where, during pregnancy, stem cells from the baby travel to the mother's body and can remain there for decades, even the entire life of the mother. What's even crazier is that in subsequent pregnancies, some of those cells can be passed along to future babies. So mothers literally carry a part of their children in the tissues of their bodies, and siblings carry each other for the rest of their lives.

Even more magical, because they're stem cells, they turn into whatever tissue they land in. So Pepper's stem cells that travel to my heart become little joy-filled Pepper heart cells inside of mine. (Also, don't scientifically fact-check this. I'm 80 percent sure I'm repeating correctly what I read. If I'm wrong, don't tell me. I prefer my interpretation.)

When they say that motherhood changes you, it literally changes you on a physiological, cellular level.

What it also means to me is that Pepper is a literal part of me. But when I say, "Pepper is a part of me," the way I would have meant it before was that *she* is a part of *me*, out there in the world. This little human that my body created and is now (almost) walking around. Some of me, out there.

So she is part me outside, but what this phenomenon shifts for me is the understanding that I am also part *her*, inside.

A few weeks ago, I was sitting in the green-velvet chair in our living room while Pepper stood on my lap, trying to pull my hair and giggling each time she got a death-grip baby handful to yank. (Side note: How do babies have the strongest grip strength on planet Earth? Do not enter into a flexed-arm-hang competition with a baby. You will lose.)

Something felt different. When our eyes met, I saw something different in her gaze. Something different about how she looked at me.

I had noticed the same thing the day before when we were playing in her "Pepper Lounge." It caught me off guard then too. It lasted a fraction of a second both times, and she instantly went back to playing, not noticing my confusion or paying any attention to me.

She was looking at me—like, really looking at me. She was having her own experience of me. I could see it in her eyes. She was thinking, observing, experiencing. In the most subtly profound way, it woke me up like a little shock when you touch a doorknob after walking across a carpeted floor.

Up until now, my entire experience of motherhood had been largely about my experience and my experience of her. When I was pregnant, although I was conscious of what I put into my body so she would be healthy, I was more present to my experience of being pregnant emotionally and physically.

Once she was born, it was about taking care of her, keeping her fed, clean, and safe, and enjoying her. Of course, I knew she was having her own experience of her life—observing, growing, and learning. I know from the work I do that we give meaning to our experiences from the moment we are born, shaping our identity and sense of the world from day one. But it didn't look like anything was happening; you couldn't really see it.

Now I can see it. It's so clear to me. The other day I picked her up from her windowsill where she sits every morning to air out her tush and greet the day with our morning song, to feed her, and she started crying. It occurred to me that she was upset that I had pulled her away from the baby-Adidas shoebox she was taking socks in and out of. I had ripped her away from her experience without warning, and she was pissed.

I felt terrible! I even apologized out loud to her—"Oh my god! I'm sorry! I didn't realize I interrupted you!"—and put her back down for a few minutes, stunned. This had never happened before. Before this moment, she went along with whatever was happening. I stared at her in slight disbelief and confusion and then asked and invited her to come with me for breakfast. She was much more willing the second time. I'm now cautious before simply scooping her up. I let her know we're relocating and give her a few seconds to process that a change is coming before tearing her away. But this is new. Like, brand new.

A few days ago, we were at a friend's house to celebrate the birthday of her one-year-old boy. Later that evening, collapsed on the couch together, Sibe said, "I have to tell you, there were some tough moments for me today. I wanted to say, 'Hey, don't fucking touch my kid. Give her toy back!'"

I laughed. He was referring to the other kids playing with her, all under the age of two.

I was more focused that day on how Pepper would handle it rather than feeling inclined to push in, while also secretly hoping she would steal the toy back herself.

But all of this—the new way she looked at me, her crying when I pulled her away from her box of socks that no longer fit, and her playing in this new environment, handling her toys being taken by another kid—showed me something both beautiful and painful.

It's not just me and P anymore.

I guess what I really mean is that it's not just me *for* P anymore. I'm not her whole world. Her world is expanding, and now I'm simply part of it.

I know this is exactly how it's supposed to work. My job is to love her, teach her to trust herself, and preserve the joy and confidence she came into this world with so that she can go out there and do whatever she came here to do. But part of me wants to just lock her up in her Pepper Lounge for the rest of her life with me. And selfishly keep that limitless little heart and those pudgy baby thighs all for myself. I don't want to share her with the world. I don't want to share her with anyone. I want to go back to the hospital the three days after she was born where Sibe and I cocooned up with lavender essential oils and soft guitar music playing in the background day and night. I want to create a force field where nothing can hurt her and no one else can have her but Sibe, Opi, and me. I want to keep every baby giggle, every toothless smile, and every ounce of that baby chub and love to myself. Forever.

I joke that, to me, pregnancy wasn't all that beautiful. It freaked me out. I felt like a host body for some alien being to grow.

Sure, I "created" her. But it really is more like I hosted a space for her to come through. And she's not mine. And as much as I want to take all of the credit and keep her all to myself, this new look in her eye, the crying when I take her away from her shoebox, lets me know that's not my job.

I thought it was my job to guide her, guard her, and teach her, this little part of me out there in the world. But I'm starting to see that that's only half of it. I'm not here to guide her the direction I think she should go.

Her tiny little stem cells micro-chromerismed their way up into my heart and merged her little Pepper heart into mine. I am also part her. I am as much a part of her as she is me, and I see that I'm not here to teach her what I think. I'm here to preserve her joy while she teaches me everything she came here already knowing.

33.

BREAK YOUR HEART OPEN
(DEAR PEPPER)

"DO YOU HEAR HER?" Sibe asked from the other room.

"What?" I asked. I couldn't hear him over the superhero show I'd recently become obsessed with.

"Mute it," he said.

I muted the TV and heard Opi snoring.

"Opi?" I asked.

"No, listen."

I tried to focus, as if to turn up the volume on whatever he was hearing.

I heard a muffled cry coming from your room. I had put you to bed two hours ago, and you never wake up once you've fallen asleep. So, I waited, paused to see what you'd do. But you started to cry harder, so I sprinted to your door.

My heart was racing. Truthfully, it was racing in part because I could hear that you were upset. And partly because I was excited to get to pick you up again so soon after putting you down.

You won't remember this, but just as I reached for your door handle, you stopped. I placed my opposite hand on the door, waiting to hear what would happen before I rushed in. I remembered a lesson from your sleep-training course: "Give babies six minutes of trying to settle themselves before you go to them."

But just then you cried again, and it sounded so sad. I pushed the door open into your dark room and saw you crying in your crib. Within seconds, I had you in my arms, your chubby cheeks wet from your tears against my cheek, and we plopped down into the big grey rocking chair in your room. The second we hit the chair, you stopped crying. You snuggled in closer to me, wrapped your chubby little leg over my knee, and put your two fingers into your mouth and fell asleep.

You stopped crying. You won't remember this, but I will. I stared at you for twenty minutes. You fell deeper and deeper into sleep, and I swear you felt bigger than when I put you down two hours before. I closed my eyes and pressed my forehead against yours and felt a tear fall down my cheek.

I was overwhelmed by love for you. It was too much for my body to hold, and it pushed its way up into my eyes and out through tears. I know it sounds insane, but I loved you so much in that moment that it felt like my heart was breaking.

As I held you closer, it felt like time was slipping away. I thought of my mom, who probably rushed in to rescue me from a bad dream and rock me to sleep hundreds of times that I'll never remember.

I was with my mom the other day and I said to her, "I realized, obvious as it may seem, that you held me like that too, a million times. You must have loved me as much as I love her. And now you must have all of these complex emotions about your kids."

"I still do love you that much," she replied. "And you have complex emotions about me too."

Our relationship, too, will get complex. I'll get mad at you someday; you'll push me away, shut me out. You'll have secrets that I don't know about. You'll judge me, and I you. Despite how much we love each other and how good we are to each other, we won't be able to escape our humanness. We'll have history, and make up meaning about it.

But at this moment, none of that has happened yet. Our love is still perfect, and I want to stop time and hold us here forever.

My heart is breaking because I know I can't stop any of it. You will grow up. We will grow up.

You took your first steps today. A day after I wrote about not rushing your evolution to walk. I put a gold measuring cup in each of your hands to help you forget about reaching for me, because I knew you could do it on your own. With your hands full, you forgot your fear and took ten steps toward your dad. Then you plopped down onto your butt and crawled after our friend's cat. We cheered and laughed, and you didn't even realize anything special was happening.

To you, it was just your evolution taking place in its own time. As joy-filled as that moment was, as happy as I was for you to be gaining independence, I couldn't believe that you're already walking. Just two weeks before your first birthday. I can't believe you're almost one. I can't believe I've been a mother for almost a year—that, in a way, I'm almost one.

Sitting in that chair, I saw you grown up, moved out, living your own life. I felt like I was forward in time, looking back on this beautiful moment. Trying to run back and relive this moment a thousand more times as it was happening.

But I couldn't. I could only live it now, as much as I could. I considered sleeping the night in your room, in that chair with you. But you started stretching out and rolling your head along my arm, a gesture that meant you were sleeping and uncomfortable, ready for your bed.

I soaked in the moment for a second longer, trying to tattoo it on my heart forever, realizing how many other moments like this I'd probably already forgotten.

I walked out of the room, placing my opposite hand on the door to close it silently. A few steps out of your room, I sat down on the couch. Your dad was sleeping with Opi. I let the tears flow. Before I knew it, I was sobbing. Crying so hard. But not sad. So absolutely overwhelmed by love that I just couldn't hold.

There is a poem by Rumi called "Heartbreak."

He wrote, "You have to keep breaking your heart until it opens."

I thought he was just writing about heartbreak. The hard stuff, the challenging moments that teach us something.

But he meant more than that. Love breaks your heart. It has to. The expansion my love creates has to break my heart. It's just not big enough to hold it all.

My sense is that the heartbreak I felt in that moment was the first of thousands. I can only hope that my love for you will grow to such impossible size that my heart will have to break over and over and over again to try to hold it. And it will never be able to. Eventually it will just open.

34.

THE PARK AT SUNRISE

I'M WRITING THIS PIECE at sunrise in the woods with Opi running around.

It's an early-June morning, and the air is slightly cool but humid and damp and warm on my arms. The birds are loud and many, and there's a sweet plant smell in the air. A mix of grass, dirt, and honeysuckle.

I feel like me. Like a version I've dreamed up a million times. The kind of person who gets up before the sun and can slow down enough to spend her mornings in the woods with her dog. Who, before she starts her workday, has already lived and enjoyed her life. And that joy radiates through her day.

I feel happy and fulfilled. And there is also a rushed feeling in my chest, and my eyes keep automatically shifting to the time on my screen. Instant math equations let me know I have forty minutes left, and even that might not be enough.

Pepper wakes up at seven, and it's ten to six. It's a fourteen-minute drive home, and I have to stop at my friend's to hose Opi down before taking her home. I'll never make it in time.

I start to feel stressed, frustrated, and rushed. I'm disappointed that I'm going to miss her waking up. And I'm equally stressed because I've committed to waking up, hiking, and writing for the next seven days. And I don't want to miss her waking up every day for a week.

I feel irritated. Almost instantly I feel trapped. Martyred. "Where is my time to be me? How will I get this done? How am I supposed to write a book, or run a business, or do anything when I constantly have a clock running out until I'm off work and back on duty?" The pressure feels intense, unfair, and impossible to change.

And for the first time, I can see the beauty in that. And then I can hear the birds again. The yellow flowers against the green grass come back into focus, and I hear Opi snorting like a truffle pig as she searches for the one weed she loves to eat.

It's beautiful. The rushed feeling. The disappointment at missing Pepper wake up.

It's actually expansion. It's love pushing against fear, asking for more room.

A year ago, I would have been sacrificing time with Pepper to write a book about Pepper, probably not missing Pepper because I would have told myself some version of "Just get the book done and you'll make up for time later when your book is a best seller and you have all the time and money in the world to spend with her."

It's sweet, isn't it? Sitting in the woods, feeling like myself, the version I've dreamed about? Writing a book about Pepper, missing Pepper?

I've slowed down. I'm starting to understand what it means to be present. And while I can't know for sure, my guess is that someday when P is older, I'll be so glad it took me so much longer to do everything because of the quality time we spent together. I already feel that way about the time we've had up until now.

It also strikes me that I, a mother (*gasps with her hand on her chest*), am sitting in the woods at sunrise. Something I've told myself I'd do a million times before and never have. I feel like the most me I've ever been. As a *mother*, the most me. Huh. Who knew?

35.

A MONK AND HIS TEACHER

A STUDENT MONK SITS with his teacher in a forest.

He says, "How do you reach enlightenment?"

The teacher sits quietly for minutes.

Right as the young monk is about to ask again, his teacher asks, "Do you hear that mountain stream?"

The student listens quietly for a few moments and says, "Yes."

The teacher replies, "Enter Zen from there."

After a little while, they begin walking. Even more time goes by before the young monk asks, "What if I hadn't heard the mountain stream? What would your answer have been then?"

The teacher answers, "Enter Zen from there."

You can reach enlightenment, access your growth, do your healing from anywhere.

I chose motherhood.

Well, I suppose motherhood chose me.

But I didn't have to use it as an access point. I could have just muscled through it like I'd done most everything in my life.

But I chose motherhood.

I had a full-body experience when I typed those words.

Up until this moment, my experience has not been consistent with that.

The way I saw it, first, I got pregnant unplanned.

Then I resisted motherhood.

Then I embraced motherhood.

Then I loved motherhood.

But wow, I chose motherhood. That feels magical and completely different.

I did. I didn't have to have a baby. I did have a choice. Only I didn't.

There was always only one choice to make. And I made that choice. But up until now, it's felt more like I chose to have a baby and the byproduct was that I also became a mother.

But choosing motherhood feels different.

I don't think I did choose motherhood initially. I think I just chose to have a baby.

But a moment ago, just as I typed those words, I chose motherhood.

I chose motherhood as a vehicle to do the work on myself and as a result came to love it.

But there was still a part of me that resisted the word, the label, and everything that came with it.

In this moment it feels so different. It feels like a holy choice.

I chose motherhood.

I *choose* motherhood.

36.

THE ENDGAME

THERE'S A SCENE AT THE END of *Avengers*: *Infinity War* where Thanos, the bad guy, who basically looks like a purplish alien thug version of Gerard Butler from *300*, is sitting by himself on his beautiful garden planet, watching the sun rise "over a grateful universe." He has just destroyed half of life in the universe with a literal snap of his fingers, his deranged plan to restore balance in an overrun system.

That's a little how I feel today. It feels like, with the snap of God's fingers, half of everything in my universe was destroyed, and I'm sitting here at sunrise, smiling over a grateful life.

Sibe is at work, Opi is snoring in my bed, and Pepper is (fingers crossed—I don't want to jinx it) still asleep. The house is quiet, my heart is quiet, and my soul is quiet. The left corner of my mouth turns up in a half smile as I feel the calm, quiet gratitude for my life and a little nostalgia and sweet disappointment at completing this journey. This book has almost become a partner in my evolution this year. I feel like Tom Hanks from *Cast Away*; my Wilson is this book. The cursor flashes on my laptop screen somewhat impatiently, waiting to know what words to put down. I meditate on the flashing cursor for a moment and wonder how I never used that as a tool to focus before.

I talked to my sister on the phone last night and we cried as I read to her from my book and then laughed with gratitude that the other one was also crying.

"I was worried about you," she said honestly when the laughter died down, "when you told me initially. But I'm in awe of who you've become through this journey."

So was I. So am I.

A year ago today, almost to the minute, I was sitting in the courtyard of the hospital on a bench, Sibe was next to me, holding my hand, and there was a man quietly and almost invisibly moving around, tending to the flowers. I was hysterical, sobbing. I don't think I'd ever cried so hard before. I was absolutely terrified. I called my mom and could barely get any words out. In the moment I thought I was terrified of labor, and I was. But I think, looking back, deeper down I knew God had snapped his fingers. I knew half of my universe was about to be destroyed, and it scared me to death.

Sitting here now, I have so much love for me in that moment. I almost wish I could go sit down next to her and tell her about everything that would unfold. I might skip the part where her actual labor is a fucking dumpster fire, but just after that, life would change in a way she could never have imagined.

I am astounded at how much Pepper has learned, grown, and developed in one year. She went from a brand-new baby who couldn't even see to a wild, joy-filled, silly spirit who loves everything, waves at the car when we get out of it, WWE slams down onto Sibe when he's sleeping, and pulls fur out of Opi's leg while we're driving, giggling mischievously in the back seat of the car when Opi huffs grumpily. And she's *one*. She won't even consciously remember anything she's learned this year. She knows *nothing* compared to what she will learn.

I am astounded at how much I have grown and developed in one year. I went from a terrified woman sobbing in a courtyard, afraid of life, both the one she lived and the one she was about to bring into the world, and who in so many ways had things *mostly* right but also profoundly wrong, to a woman who takes dance breaks between coaching calls, is finally learning to prioritize social connection over productivity, hikes at sunrise with her dog, writes books, snuggles her daughter 1,000 times a day, and *really* loves her husband. My heart feels limitless. In so many ways I feel like I have this down. I'll hold while you laugh. And yet, I am also one. I have *so* much growing to do. I know even less than Pepper about parenting at this age. I know nothing compared to what I will learn.

Up until this very moment, I was still really upset about the way Pepper's birth unfolded. It felt so deeply unfair to have been unconscious for it. I experienced that as missing the transition from not-mother to mother. In this moment I see it differently. I needed to be unconscious. I don't think I actually woke up from that surgery. My shaman referred to it once as a "rescue mission." That it was heading south, fast, and one or both of us weren't going to make it out of there.

Sitting here now, feeling how I feel, I'm pretty sure I didn't. Half of me didn't, anyway—the me who was sitting in the courtyard crying. I think she knew she was going to die. That's why she was so afraid. God snapped his fingers. She knew.

It's *almost* too cliché to say, but Pepper's birthday was the first day of my life. The delivery wasn't a dumpster fire; it was a forest fire, clearing away everything that was suffocating the growth and expansion of the forest. To make space for my life. My *real* life, my growth, the real me. This real me has a limitless heart. My love is infinite. I have the capacity to love the whole world.

Happy birthday, Pepper.

Your birthday. My birth day.

We are one.

EPILOGUE
ME

IT NEVER CEASES TO AMAZE me how different it feels to be away from Pepper for a few days. The amount of energy that pours into that tiny little human just absolutely blows my mind. It's always after her first night away from home that I realize just how tired I have actually been and remind myself not to wait two more months to do this again.

Our week started with me asking Sibe on Monday at 9 a.m. if he thought it was too early to start drinking. I recalled my insight from a few weeks prior that reminded me to acknowledge my needs and ask for help before I got to a state where I was convinced I was the only human on earth who cared about Pepper and had an existential crisis about the idea that absolutely no one cared about me. Instead, I called my mom and asked her to take P for the weekend, to which she enthusiastically agreed.

Sibe kept saying that he was "just so surprised" that I did that. That it "just came out of nowhere." I later realized that this was probably the first time I had ever just acknowledged my needs and asked for help without first having a breakdown, and Sibe was totally unfamiliar with that experience.

By Thursday, I can't recall that I actually did one thing that was useful aside from a few great coaching conversations with clients, a sum total of four hours of work. Thursday at 2 p.m., I cracked a beer with my good friend mid-run when we realized one of our favorite riverside bars was open as we passed it on the trail.

By Saturday afternoon, we were feeling more relaxed, but laughed because we spent half the day preparing for Pepper's birthday party the following weekend.

"Even when Pepper's not here, it's all about Pepper," Sibe joked. By Sunday morning, I felt like me again.

Initially, when Pepper started to develop her own sense of independence, I felt sad. I wanted to slow down her growth and keep her to myself, completely dependent and attached to me. But as that fiery and mischievous look in her eye shows up more and more often—the look that says, "You do you, Mom. I'm going my own way"—I see that when I let the subtle sadness settle for a few seconds, what's left is me. As Pepper claims her independence, it creates space for me to do the same.

This entire journey over the past year has had me so focused on who I am becoming and what I'm learning in relation to motherhood and my marriage that it's only recently occurred to me to slow down and acknowledge who I have become as an individual.

Hardly the me that threw that pregnancy test under the bathroom sink and somehow made it through a two-hour coaching call immediately after. Certainly not the me that had multiple breakdowns over the crushing weight of losing my entire sense of identity and achievement.

Although my life has become more rooted, and I am completely attached logistically and energetically now to Pepper and, even more deeply, to Sibe, I feel more me—more free and more independent than I've ever felt. To others who don't know me that well, I might not seem that different. To those who know me well, I am very different. To myself, I am unrecognizable.

Four months into my pregnancy, I went to have my yearly tarot reading. I had been crying the entire day. I had been part letting it out, part laughing about it with Sibe, and part holding it in. I sat down in the chair in the tiny back room lit with a small lamp, a pretty lace curtain, and crystals on the table in front of me. We hadn't even begun yet and I just fell apart.

Part tarot reader, part medium, the same woman who had told me the month before I discovered I was pregnant that my womb was getting ready for a baby, Leslie sat there, deck of cards in hand. "This child is coming to heal you," she said after a few patient moments.

My mind shot to a few weeks prior. Just after announcing our pregnancy to the family, my mom had a dream. In it, she received the message: "A healer is coming."

I didn't think of myself as a person who needed healing. Though a coach myself, I thought of myself as a person who was tough, brave, strong, and independent. A person who needed to apply those traits more often and more consistently and intensely to her life. But I was a person who desperately needed healing.

A few years prior to that, a good friend looked me in the eye and said, "Put the world down, Vanessa. Your soul is tired of carrying it."

I had been receiving this message for years, and yet I couldn't seem to put the world down, stop running, or stop trying to achieve more. And I was tired; my soul was tired. Of running, of trying, of controlling. I was so tired of being me, but I just couldn't trust any other way of being. Even if I had, I had no idea how to get there.

As I sit here, a few days before Pepper's first birthday, that me is almost a ghost. I remember her, and I feel her echo sometimes. I remember my shaman's words early in my pregnancy: "This pregnancy is a gift. Your current identity structure is too small. It lacks spiritual depth. This pregnancy is a gift from God to break apart your old identity structure so that you can create a new one that is big enough for who you really are."

When I lived in Perth, Western Australia, I used to take Bikram yoga classes three times a week. The level of strength and flexibility in my body was unbelievable. I went from nearly passing out during my first class to enjoying the ninety minutes in 105-degree heat as a rejuvenating, quick morning routine. But locust pose, an awkward posture where you lie on your stomach with your arms extended under your body, palms on the floor, chin extended, and you lift both legs off the ground at the same time, was nearly impossible. Despite coming three times a week, I couldn't even get my toes to hover. I brought it to the attention of my instructor after class one day and she said simply, "The postures you hate the most are the ones you most need."

I find that to be true of most things in life. The thing you most resist is the thing you most need. So, it's no surprise that motherhood, the thing I was sure would be the end of me, destroy my life, and condemn me to a life I'd resent, was the very thing I most needed. The thing that would in fact end me—a version of me I was sick of but couldn't outrun. The thing that would destroy my life, a life that wasn't even what I wanted. That would change how I experienced that life and set me free to live the life I had been trying to live all along but didn't know how.

It's interesting. I'm so much more comfortable calling myself a mother. Using the word *motherhood*. I don't even have to say to myself anymore, "I am Pepper's mom." I can simply say, "I am a mom." Sibe and I have even talked about names for another tiny human in the next few years. But I don't *feel* like a mom, a mother, the way I used the word before I became one.

I thought I'd end up a MOTHER, this massive identity that swallowed and imprisoned the real me to the depths of the smallest Russian stacking doll. But I just feel like me. I feel like the *real* me. The me-est me there ever was, the one who had been locked up, unable to experience life, trapped behind another version of myself I created by accident. And I guess the real me is also a mother. But "mom" is an aspect of a much bigger me. Like an arm, not a shadow.

I can see so much of the beauty, complexity, and sacredness of motherhood. I can also see all of the ideas that I had about it, both self-generated and conditioned, and I see how many women get swallowed by it, or lost in it, or even choose it as their life's purpose.

Everything has changed for me over the past year and nine months. Initially, the deepest parts of me were shaken alive. The masked parts had to be shed. And layer by layer, anything that wasn't the real me has fallen away, from the deepest, hidden, inside layers out.

The outer layers are now also starting to shift, literally. I emptied my closet with my visual branding coach the other day. There probably aren't more than twenty total items left hanging there. The rest were remnants of a muted version of me, and they had to go. We're starting the rebuild this week. Edgy, elegant, and wild.

We're planning a move to Colorado in the fall, to confirm our intuition that this city in the middle of the mountains will be our new home. Trading in city streets for rocky trails and eating out for exploring outside. Muted city tones for awesome landscapes. Everything that isn't me is getting left behind.

For most of my adult life, I've had a vision of myself that has been painful to behold. Painful because she felt impossible to touch, my life impossibly far from hers. This version of me is always happy, always smiling; her body is fit because of her connection to her life. She's always doing the same thing in the vision. She's unpacking her Jeep Wrangler with gear she's used on her weekend trip hiking, camping, and spending time in the water. She's with a small group of close friends and Sibe after an awesome weekend of exploring, music coming out of the speakers of the car, and they're about to sit down at a beat-up white plastic table on the beach, open a Corona, and she's about to stick her feet in the sand. She's happy, so content.

She's absolutely her, the most authentic, real her. There's nothing about her, on her, or around her that isn't a complete DNA match.

There's just a part of this vision that wasn't visible to me before. She's got a backpack on, with someone in the back—a complete DNA match.

ACKNOWLEDGMENTS

THE PHRASE "IT TAKES A VILLAGE" has taken on completely new meaning in the creation of this book, the creation of a tiny human, and the recreation of myself.

First, my husband, Sibe. Aside from allowing me to share some of our most intimate details with the world, you celebrate and support my vulnerability, and challenge me to be more authentic and to constantly live into higher expressions of my integrity. Despite— and perhaps even more so—when I am kicking and screaming, you lovingly hold me to the highest version of myself.

To my own parents. I remember the exact moment that I realized you were people before you were parents. And I learned what that really means when I became one myself. The level of selflessness, grace, and humility you have shown over the years blows my mind. Especially you, Mom, in the honest writing of this book and healing of my own wounds. You graciously continue to hold space to allow me my experience. And each time I move through it, I have more respect, adoration, and love for you.

To my sisters. Increasing levels of humility are required as I recognize how many of my flaws you silently witnessed, how you have seen my blind spots and lovingly allowed me to fumble around in my ego as you knew I would not be open to hearing about them. Thank you for loving me, supporting me, and being on this journey with me. If I could choose you all over again, I would.

To my coaches, John Patrick Morgan, Kamin Samuel, Steve Chandler, and Devon Bandison, thank you for ceaselessly holding a space to release my "accidental" personality and for providing the wisdom, support, and encouragement to create the one I want intentionally. Thank you for refusing to believe my stories, calling me out relentlessly, offering possibility where I saw none, and teaching me the true meaning of loving, selfless service.

To my shaman, Patrick Carroll. It's no understatement to say that you helped save my life—more specifically, my experience of myself in my life. Thanks to our work together, I have the capacity to be fully in love and present with my daughter, free of resentment, pressure, and struggle. Of the countless moments I spend snuggling her, totally lost in love, my gratitude for you shows up in so many of them. Thank you for showing me who I really am and reminding me that outside of this moment, we are eternal, spiritual beings.

To my many friends and teachers in the coaching world and outside. Thank you for loving me, celebrating my life with me, and for continually reminding me of what I often forget, pass over, and take for granted. As I move into the next phase of my life, your friendships mean increasingly more to me, and my definition of success has simplified to "be a more present and loving friend."

To my publisher and editors, thank you for believing in my project, taking me under your wing, and cultivating me as a professional in this craft. Your guidance, humor, and wisdom are deeply appreciated.

And to Pepper. Thank you, beyond what words could ever express, for coming into my life exactly as you did, when you did.

Thank you for making me a mother, choosing me as your mother, and continuing to be the greatest teacher I will ever know. I vow to you to preserve your beautiful spirit, allow you to expand through all of your life's experiences, and to do my best to provide you an infinite space of love, safety, and trust to always be exactly who you are and love you more and more for it. You are truly the most remarkable soul I have ever met, and I am honored to support you on your journey. You have taught me more about love than I could have ever wished to learn. And you're only one.

To learn more about Vanessa and her work, visit:

www.vanessabroerscoaching.com
https://vanessabroerscoaching.medium.com/
Friend her 'Vanessa Broers' on facebook
Follow her on instagram @vanessabroerscoaching

And most preferred, email her directly at vanessa@
vanessabroerscoaching.com to share what you took from reading
this book, to say hello or just connect. (She's a real person and
responds to every email.)

Lightning Source UK Ltd.
Milton Keynes UK
UKHW010625180821
389030UK00001B/99